TOP ATHLETES AND EXPERTS PRAISE...

THE 12-MINUTE TOTAL-BODY WORKOUT

"AN EXCELLENT WORKOUT...not just for beginners, but for bodybuilders who want to maintain their physiques while on the road for weeks at a time and unable to get to a gym. I can see where this workout would not only keep every muscle hard, tight and 'ripped,' but would make 'starting up again' in the gym seem like a breeze because the muscles were not left dormant."
–Robert Kennedy,
  bestselling author of *Rock Hard,*
  Hardcore Bodybuilding, and *Pumping Up*

"BY FAR THE SAFEST METHOD OF WORKING OUT I'VE EVER SEEN."
–Jack Barnathan, Doctor of Chiropractic,
  Director, Sports Health Chiropractic and
  Chiropractic Health Care Consultant to the
  Miss Olympia Contest

"WHENEVER A BEGINNER OR NONEXERCISER ASKS ME HOW TO GET STARTED, I ALWAYS ANSWER: 'GET ONE OF JOYCE VEDRAL'S BOOKS.'"
–Rochelle Larkin,
  Editor-in-Chief,
  Female Bodybuilding & Weight Training magazine

"JOYCE VEDRAL HAS COME UP WITH TOTAL-BODY ISOMETRICS. IT'S EASY TO FOLLOW. IT'S FUN. IT WORKS!"
–Cameo Kneuer,
  Miss National Fitness and Hostess for
  E.S.P.N. American Muscle Magazine Television Show

"GREAT FOR SHAPING AND TONING THE BODY. A GUIDELINE FOR A LIFETIME OF WORRY-FREE EATING!"
–Joe Weider,
  Trainer of Champions and Publisher of
  Muscle and Fitness, Flex, Sports Fitness,
  and *Shape* magazines

"EXCELLENT BEFORE A CONTEST! Anyone who follows this workout will get peak muscle performance, peak muscle shape, and peak muscle separation."
–Gus Stefanidis,
  a Personal Trainer and Mr. Greece

"THE BEGINNING OF A NEW ERA IN EXERCISING...an excellent way of toning and defining your body, for that shapely new look."
–Andy Silvert,
  Owner, Mr. America's Fitness Center and
  First Runner-Up, Mr. America

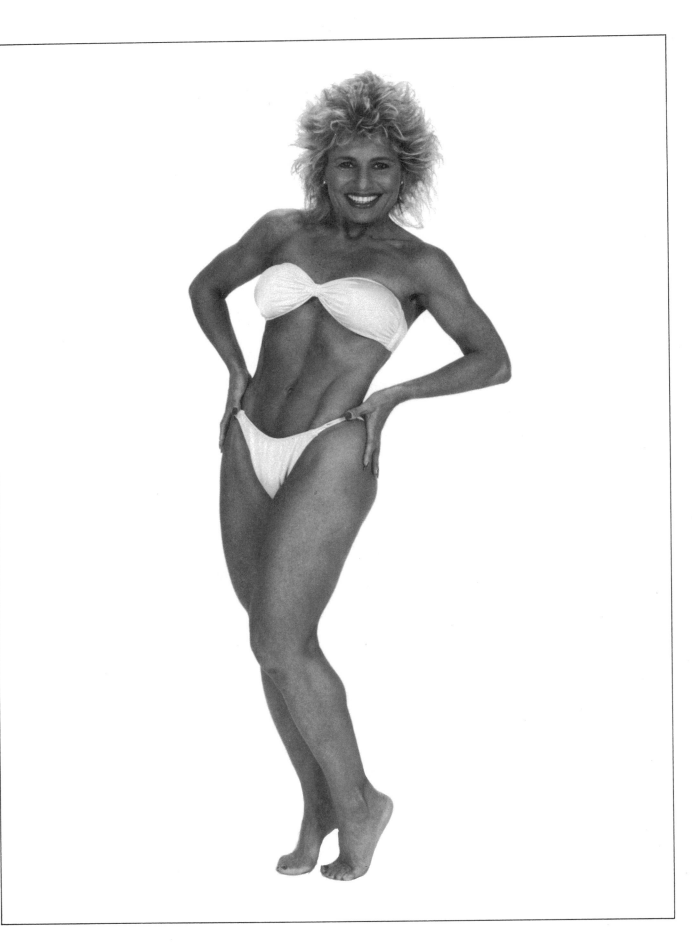

THE
12-MINUTE
TOTAL-BODY
WORKOUT

JOYCE L. VEDRAL, Ph.D.

WARNER BOOKS

A Time Warner Company

Warner Books, Inc., 1271 Avenue of the Americas, New York, NY 10020

W A Time Warner Company

Printed in the United States Of America
First printing: February 1989
10 9 8 7

Library of Congress Cataloging-in-Publication Data

Vedral, Joyce L.
  The 12-minute total-body workout.

  1. Exercise. I. Title. II. Title: Twelve-minute
total-body workout.
GV481.V42 1988   613.7′1   88-14331
  ISBN 0-446-38961-7 (pbk.)

A NOTE FROM THE PUBLISHER
The ideas, procedures, and suggestions contained in this book are not intended as a substitute for consulting with your physician. All matters regarding your health require medical supervision.

Book design by Richard Oriolo
Cover design by Jackie Merri Meyer
Cover photo by Don Banks
Black-and-white photos by Don Banks
Hair and Makeup by Diane Matthews
Cover bathing suit by Just Bikinis Inc. by Joyce Holder
Workout leotard by Capezio® from Ballet Makers, Inc.
Ballet slippers by Capezio® from Ballet Makers, Inc.
Leg warmers by Capezio® from Ballet Makers, Inc.
Gym shoes by Reebok International Ltd.

MENUS:
The Westin Bonaventure, Los Angeles, California
Pittsburgh Green Tree Marriott
Omni International Hotel, Detroit
Holiday Inn–Runnemede, New Jersey

To those of us who, in spite of a hectic schedule,
insist upon having a tight, toned, sensual body, and who are willing
to invest 12 minutes a day in that project.

And to Randie Levine and Sandi Kopler,
sophisticated ladies with a
great sense of humor.

ACKNOWLEDGMENTS

To Joann Davis, my astute, sensitive editor, for your wisdom and wit.

To Jackie Merri Meyer, for your loving attention and creative art direction on the cover and photography of the book.

To Larry Kirshbaum, Nansey Neiman, Ling Lucas, and Ellen Herrick, for your belief in this project.

To my agent, Rick Balkin, for your continual guidance and confidence.

To all the women who experimented with this program, and who achieved dramatic results.

To *Senseis* Vinnie DeMarco, Master Chang, and Hero Yamashita, for teaching me the nuances of various aspects of the martial arts.

To Joe Weider, for inventing and teaching the basic principles of body shaping, and for your wonderful magazines, *Muscle and Fitness, Shape,* and *Flex.*

To Dr. Jack Barnathan, of Bethpage, Long Island, for your excellent chiropractic advice concerning safe weight-training techniques.

To my family and friends, who are ready and willing to try new ideas.

To Uncle Dave, for transforming your body into perfect form, and for maintaining your physique.

To Sheila Melfe and Nola Roeper of WPIX "Best Talk in Town," for belief in my fitness techniques and for your delightful show.

To Bob Oskam, for your last-minute review of the manuscript to ensure the details were all properly given.

PREFACE

As a medical doctor and a participant in the martial arts, I am particularly impressed with Joyce Vedral's *12-Minute Total-Body Workout*. In it, she has created a system that is safe, simple, and at the same time effective.

The program outlined in this book, when followed exactly, will give the individual a hard, tight body rather than an overly muscular, bulky body. By using the basic principles of bodybuilding and combining them with the energy-efficient use of isometrics and dynamic tension utilized by martial artists, Vedral has created a system that will cause not only an increase in muscle tone but a marked improvement in posture and general energy level.

For many years, those of us who have practiced the martial arts have used what is called "dynamic tension" in the performance of our basic movements. It is the use of dynamic tension, the continual pressure on the muscle when performing a particular movement, that causes the muscle to strengthen, harden, and become "tight" as opposed to flaccid. Strength and muscle tone are thus created, not by the use heavy weights, but by the continual tension on the muscle. *The 12-Minute Total-Body Workout* utilizes dynamic tension. For this reason, nothing more than the proscribed set of three-pound dumbbells is required to get results. Not only is this an asset when it comes to prevention of potential injury, but it is also conducive to workout continuity, because individuals will not be tempted to "lay off" when away from home. There's no reason why they can't carry the dumbbells with them. They can thus achieve and maintain a fit body no matter how much traveling they do.

What is also appealing to me about this program, is its emphasis on what is often called "interval training." Vedral presents a special "burning it up double time" plan for those who wish to get rid of excess fat as quickly as possible—without the drawback of exhausting lengthy runs, swims or walks. She presents a variety of options for 12-minute "aerobic spurts." One is able to speed up one's metabolism more efficiently by performing, for example, three separate 12-minute "exercise spurts" during the course of the day than by performing one ongoing exercise session of 36 minutes.

All things considered, I feel that Joyce Vedral's *12-Minute Total-Body Workout* would be the best 12 minutes a day anyone could hope to invest in fitness, and, in addition, it is the safest, most efficient body-toning and shaping program I have ever seen.

–JUDE T. BARBERA, M.D.
Assistant Clinical Professor of Surgery
Downstate Medical Center
Associate Director of Urology
Coney Island Hospital
Fourth Degree Black Belt Go-Ju Karate

INTRODUCTION

Most people would love to be in great shape, but the fact is, many people hesitate to begin a fitness program because they fear it will consume too much of their time. Another thing that stops many from embarking on a shape-up program is the fear that they will become overly muscular.

In her *12-Minute Total-Body Workout*, Joyce Vedral has solved these two problems. The Weider Principles of muscle isolation and the split routine can be used not only to build size and bulk, but also for muscle shaping and toning. In this book, Joyce has combined my time-tested principles with isotension to create a program for those who want to tighten and tone, rather than build large muscles. The individual following this program and exercising only 12 minutes a day will have worked the entire body twice in a week: chest, shoulders, triceps, legs, back, biceps and calves, and the troublesome buttocks and abdominals three times. Joyce also includes a "speed-up" program where she demonstrates the use of the Weider Principles of giant setting and supersetting to accelerate progress.

Without proper nutrition, however, workout efforts will be sabotaged because fat would cover the developing muscles. Therefore, the inclusion of a special chapter on how to eat at home, on the run, or anywhere in the world and maintain proper nutrition is more than helpful; it is crucial. For years I have taught champion bodybuilders not to fear food, but to enjoy it by controlling it and using it to their nutritional advantage. In her book, Joyce has done the same for the person desiring a fit body with a minimum of body fat. She takes the reader through a step-by-step plan, even going so far as to show them how to select foods from a wide variety of hotel and restaurant menus.

Not only is this book great for shaping and toning the body, and as a guideline for a lifetime of worry-free eating, but for those who eventually wish to go further, it is an excellent introduction to the basic movements and principles of bodybuilding.

—JOE WEIDER,
trainer of champions since 1936;
Publisher: "Muscle and Fitness,"
"Flex," "Sports Fitness," and
"Shape" magazines

CONTENTS

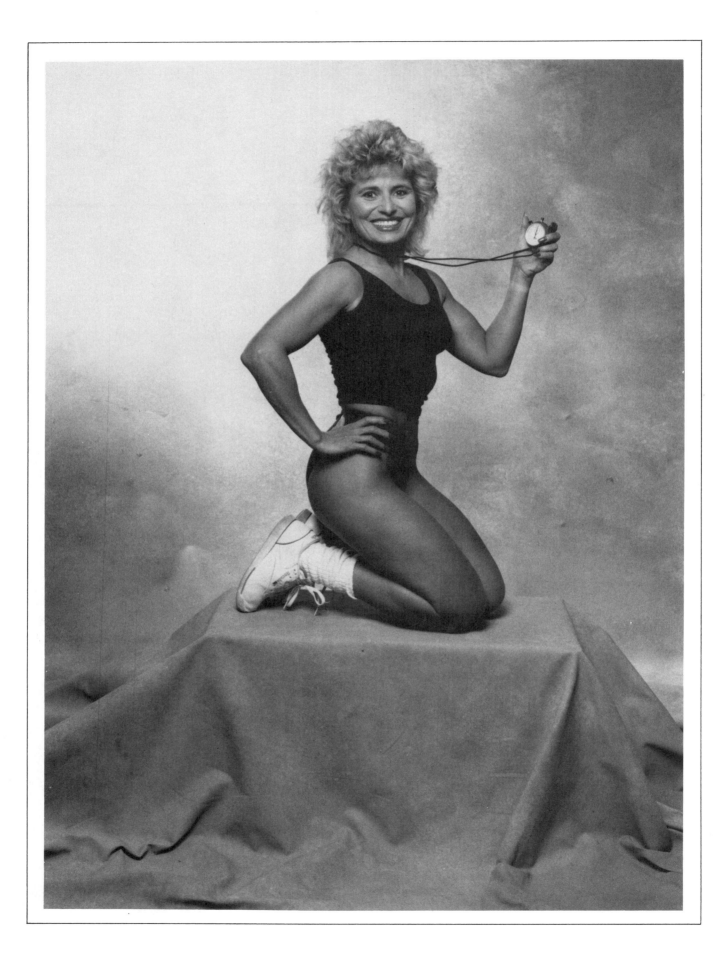

1

ONLY 12 MINUTES A DAY: WHY THIS PROGRAM WORKS

What? An exercise plan that tightens, tones, and shapes the entire body in only 12 minutes a day?—and you see results in only three weeks? Impossible, you say. Well, it really can be done, and here's why.

When it comes to body shaping (which is actually the scientific development of small muscles in all the right places), *more is not always better*. Precision *is* always better because it saves wasted time and energy. If you want to get in shape, or if you want to maintain your already shapely body, and you have very little time to invest, this program is for you. Your total commitment is *12 minutes a day*. That's it.

YOU WON'T GET BIG MUSCLES, YOU'LL GET TIGHT AND TONED

Have you ever noticed that people who engage in the martial arts such as Karate, Kung-Fu, or Tai-Chi have hard, tight bodies with well-defined small muscles—muscles much less bulky than those of hardcore bodybuilders?

Having been an active member of both groups (see About the Author, at the end of the book), I have discovered how to combine the two methods—dynamic tension and isometric pressure used by martial artists, and the movements and principles of bodybuilding—in order to produce a simple program that if followed exactly, will result in a firm, fit, symmetrical body with small, shapely muscles in all the right places.

Don't become alarmed. This program is not going to involve you in the martial arts, nor will you be required to lift heavy weights. Instead you will apply the basic principles of each "art" in order to achieve the best of both disciplines and build esthetically appealing, normal-size muscles that are perfectly formed and well placed on your particular body. You will become tight and toned, but not overly muscular. *The only equipment needed is a pair of three-pound dumbbells.*

WHY THIS PROGRAM WORKS

The program is based upon basic principles that have been used by champion bodybuilders for many years: *muscle isolation, the split routine,* and *peak contraction.* A fourth principle, the pyramid system, will not be used in this program because it requires the use of graduated weights and produces muscles somewhat larger than many people want. Our use of isometrics and dynamic tension allow self-created and self-controlled resistance. The need for any weight higher than a three-pound dumbbell is thus eliminated.

WHY THIS WORKOUT
IS UNIQUE

1. The only equipment needed is a pair of three-pound dumbbells.

2. Although you will only be working out 12 minutes a day, you'll be exercising your entire body two times a week (except buttocks and abdominals, which for reasons explained later will be exercised three times a week).

3. You can do this workout anytime and anywhere: at home, in a hotel room, a college dorm, etc.

4. A fat-burning "eat anywhere" diet is provided.

WHAT CAN YOU EXPECT FROM THIS PROGRAM?

1. A total-body workout: abdominals, buttocks, thighs, calves, biceps, triceps, chest, shoulders, and back.

2. Replacement of soft, flabby body parts with toned, symmetrical, perfectly formed body parts—with visible results in only three weeks.

3. Improved posture and walk.

4. Renewed energy.

5. A diet that will provide a lifetime release from the fear of food. (You will be able to eat in any restaurant, anywhere in the world, without breaking your diet, and you will be able to eat "on the run," at home, or out—wherever you are.

6. A lifetime eating plan where, once you have achieved your ideal body shape, you can eat anything you want, all day long once a week and on holidays and special occasions.

7. An improved self-image and more confidence in your ability to achieve goals, as you see how your consistent, daily investment of 12 minutes has transformed your body.

HOW THIS PROGRAM WAS DISCOVERED

You may have recognized me. I'm the same Joyce Vedral who traveled around the country appearing on national and local television shows, talking about my book *Now or Never,* a best-selling weight-training book for women of all ages. The *Now or Never* program requires four 75-minute sessions a week, and uses various barbells, dumbbells, and machines.

While the workout I propose in that book has been proven to be highly effective (I'm still getting thank-you letters from women whose bodies have been transformed), I discovered that many women are unable to invest the four 75-minute time blocks required to achieve results. They would rather work out every day, but in shorter spurts. In addition, many women say that they don't want to lift heavy weights because they don't want to become overly muscular. They also want a workout that requires little or no equipment—one that can be done anywhere or anytime—late at night, during baby's nap, in hotel rooms when on business trips, etc.

At the same time I was considering these requests, I was on the road myself, for weeks at a time, promoting my book. As luck would have it, I was forced to face the very problem some of the women had raised. I discovered that very often when I arrived at a hotel, the gym was closed. Even when a hotel gym was still open, I sometimes found I wasn't in the mood to put on workout clothing and race off to do my routines. As a matter of fact, I didn't want to see anyone at all. I wanted to hide in my room and just relax. Later, after unwinding, I would crave a workout. I began to wish there was something I could do in the privacy of my room—in my underwear if I so desired. What's more, I began to feel more than a little disgust when my body seemed to start saying, I am lazy and I'm getting soft. I was in trouble—I thought; I'm promoting a fitness book and I'm beginning to feel out of shape.

A combination of the survival instinct and creative improvisation took over. Since I had a pair of three-pound dumbbells with me (I needed them as props to demonstrate exercises on television), I thought, Why not devise a total-body workout using just the three-pound dumbbells? But there was one problem. The dumbbells alone would be too light to achieve the results attained with the assistance of barbells and machines. Then I remembered my father, an extremely fit and muscular man who had never lifted a weight in his life, and who told me long ago, "All you need is isometric movements that let your muscles work in resistance to each other." I then recalled the methods I had been taught in the martial arts when we performed our Katas, a series of movements designed to simulate fighting gestures. In these Katas one had to move slowly and use "dynamic tension," an isometric-type movement utilizing self-created resistance on the extension or stretch part of a body movement.

I went to work. That evening I created exercises for my entire body, combining the three-pound dumbbells with a combination of dynamic tension and bodybuilding movements—modifying and inventing as I went along. When I finished, a little more than an hour later, I was exhausted and at the same time exhilarated. Every muscle fiber in my body felt alive. What's more, I had perspired more than I had in any gym workout, and I was tired. But a beautiful feeling of relaxation took over my entire being. I felt strong, powerful, and sensual—and I slept deeply and peacefully that night.

The next night I tried to do the same thing, but my body rebelled. It wouldn't cooperate. I wasn't ready to do all that work again. That's when I remembered a basic body-shaping principle, that muscles need at least 48 hours to totally recover from a workout. So I rested that night and was determined to work again the next night.

But then I had a different idea. Why not break up the workout so that the entire body would be worked twice a week, and the buttocks and abdominals would be worked three times a week, as is required in *Now or Never* and most other standard bodybuilding books? So I set to work and invented a routine and followed it for the next three weeks. When I returned to the gym, something strange happened. Instead of feeling out of it, my muscles behaved as if they had never missed a workout, and the next day, instead of experiencing the soreness that usually follows a layoff, I felt fine. But most important, I actually missed the new workout. I felt as if something were missing in the gym workout—and it seemed as if my muscles were not being challenged to their maximum ability. I also realized how much "cheating" I had been doing—because working with the heavier weights did not allow me to completely control my movements, or to flex my muscles to maximum ability. I've been doing my new 12-minute workout ever since. Now, if you see me in a gym, I will either be working with feather-light weights and performing, in essence, this workout, or I will be experimenting with other weight-training programs.

WHAT'S THE CATCH?

You are still skeptical. You wonder how a five-hour-a-week program (as contained in *Now or Never*) can be condensed into less than an hour and a half a week. The explanation is simple—what you sacrifice in quantity you gain in quality.

- You work much more intensely—so you need do only half the amount of exercises per session. Instead of doing four exercises per body part, you do two.

- You don't waste time continually changing weights and machines. Your three-pound dumbbells are all you need.

- Because the method requires intensity, you rest only 5 to 10 seconds between sets instead of the usual 45 to 60 seconds.

- You work faster with this method. Once you get the hang of it, and are not in danger of sacrificing quality for speed, you perform each repetition just a little bit faster than you would perform a repetition with heavier weights.

- Since you are exercising every day, you only have to work on three body parts per session—not five to eight, as in most other three- or four-day bodybuilding programs.

In summary, what would otherwise take a minimum of five hours a week takes under an hour and a half a week. What would otherwise require four 75-minute sessions requires seven 12-minute sessions, because you are now working at peak efficiency with a program consisting of isometric movement, peak contraction, dynamic tension, muscle isolation, and the split routine.

THE ISOMETRIC MOVEMENT

An isometric exercise is one in which one set of muscles is briefly tensed in opposition to another set of muscles, or in opposition to a solid surface. Try it with your right biceps muscle. (For location of biceps muscle, see anatomy photo on page 31.) Sit in a chair. Isolate your biceps by pinning your upper arm to your body and extending your arm straight down at your side. Keep your elbow riveted to your waist area. Now clench your fist and squeeze (flex) your biceps muscle as hard as possible. Begin curling your arm upward, keeping the full force of the squeezing pressure on your biceps muscle. Continue to curl your arm upward until your fist reaches shoulder height. Then, continuing to squeeze your biceps muscle as hard as possible, return to the downward (start) position. Do this ten times. You have just proven that you are capable of performing this workout. (If you have trouble picturing this exercise, turn to page 75 for a photograph of start and finish positions). Notice that the muscle bulges on the upward movement. This position is ordinarily called the "flexed" position.

You've probably heard someone ask a muscular man, "Let me see you flex." Usually, the man will raise both arms above his head, clench his fists, and lower his arms into two reverse "Ls" as he squeezes his biceps as hard as possible. (This is called the "double biceps" position in bodybuilding lingo.) *Peak contraction* is realized at the point where the man (or any individual, for that matter) exerts the most "squeeze" pressure when flexing the muscle.

DYNAMIC TENSION

You will remember that in the above description, you were asked to continue to squeeze your biceps muscle as hard as possible as you extended your arm downward from the curl position. Ordinarily, it is in the down or "stretch" position of a bodybuilding exercise that most bodybuilders relax the tension on the muscle. In fact, traditional weight-training manuals instruct the exerciser to get a full stretch and to slightly relax on the down position. The basic difference between the 12-minute total-body workout and a traditional bodybuilding workout is the use of *dynamic tension.* When you use dynamic tension, you continue to flex—harder than ever—through the down or stretch position. But, you may think, that is a contradiction, is it not? After all, how can one flex a muscle when it is being elongated or stretched. Isn't it impossible to flex while stretching or elongating? No. Not if pressure or tension is applied to the muscle. This active force of keeping the pressure on the muscle as it is elongated is called dynamic tension—energetic, forceful power in motion. Since this pressure is applied on the stretch movement, it is called tension. (The word *tension* comes from the Latin root *tensio,* to stretch.) There's power in tension—especially if you apply it with energy and force in motion. You are the dynamo—the mover who decides how taut that muscle will be as it is elongated, stretched, or tensed.

MUSCLE ISOLATION

The second secret to this program is that of muscle isolation. Champion bodybuilders have been using this training principle for years—a method in which each muscle of the body is exercised individually, in isolation from most other muscles. Muscle isolation is not achieved in an activity such as walking. When you walk you exercise many muscles at the same time. You work your thighs, calves, shoulders, pectorals, abdominals, buttocks, and even your neck and your back. That's why walking is one of the best exercises for reducing overall body fat, but not for reshaping specific parts of your body.

In contrast, when you perform an isolation exercise, you work on only one body part—and you can ultimately reshape that body part. For example, if you do a side lateral raise for your shoulders (see page 87), you exercise only your side shoulder (deltoid) muscles. No other muscles are significantly involved.

Another requirement of muscle isolation is that you perform all exercises for a given body part in sequence. For example, it is not okay to do one shoulder exercise, then one abdominal exercise, and then go back to a shoulder exercise. All shoulder exercises must be completed before moving to the next body part—triceps, for example. Then all triceps exercises must be completed before moving to the next body part, and so on. (The only exception to this rule is when you "superset" or "giant-set." See Chapter 9 for details.)

Muscle isolation is necessary for maximum muscle growth. If you jump around from one body part to another, the muscles are not challenged for the length of time required for muscle growth and development. Muscles, after all, respond to the demand being made upon them. If a muscle "realizes" that it will soon be given a break, it will not grow stronger, bigger, and harder. If it is made to understand, on the other hand, that it will have to keep up a steady pace of work, it will literally rise to the occasion.

Muscle isolation is practiced, unwittingly, in various sports. Notice the forearm of the hitting hand of a tennis player, or the thighs (quadriceps) of a soccer player. These individuals are continually isolating those specific muscles in order to play their sport. Bodybuilding aside, it's too bad there is no existing sport that isolates all the muscles and works them evenly so that each muscle is as impressively developed as a tennis player's forearm. My 12-minute total-body workout is designed to accomplish what the art of bodybuilding can achieve, only without the "baggage" of bodybuilding, without the weights, benches, machines, etc.

THE SPLIT ROUTINE

The third secret of this program is the split routine. Because muscles need at least 48 hours to recover from a workout (they use that time to grow in strength, size, and density), it is inadvisable to work the same muscles two days in a row. If you ignore this basic rule and train the same muscles every day, you will be guilty of *overtraining* them. When this happens, you are literally taking one step forward and half a step backward; the end result is little muscular improvement and a lot of weariness, boredom, and disappointment.

When I first started working out, I thought the more the better, so I exercised my entire body two hours a day, six days a week. I looked better than I would have looked if I had done nothing at all, but not nearly as good as I do now—training the correct way and putting in a mere fraction of the time. You don't always have to work harder to look better. You have to work smarter.

If you were planning to work out only four times a week, you would have to split your routine into halves—working one half of the body (or four to five body parts) on each workout day. But since you are working out seven days a week, you only have to work three body parts a day. Here's what your split routine will look like:

MONDAY: Chest, shoulders, triceps
TUESDAY: Thighs, buttocks, abdominals
WEDNESDAY: Back, biceps, calves
THURSDAY: Chest, shoulders, triceps
FRIDAY: Thighs, buttocks, abdominals
SATURDAY: Back, biceps, calves
SUNDAY: Buttocks, abdominals

(Details will be given in Chapters 4 through 9, describing each workout day. Skip around and see for yourself how simple it will be to do.)

Notice that you will be working each body part two times a week, except for buttocks and abdominals, which require an extra weekly workout. These stubborn body parts are the areas where fat tends to accumulate on most people. (Men usually major in "gut," while women major in "butt.")

TO MAKE A LONG STORY SHORT

For the sake of brevity, the entire workout given above can be summarized in the simple phrase "the ID system," because it uniquely combines isometric pressure and dynamic tension in a framework of basic body-shaping techniques.

WORKOUT BOREDOM

You will be doing different exercises each day—even on days when you perform your second weekly workout for that body part. I could have asked you to repeat your exercises on those days, and you would still have gotten into shape, but I didn't—for two reasons: (1) Your muscles will respond best to a variety of exercises that demand each muscle work from slightly different angles each time; (2) a variety of exercises prevents boredom and the temptation to skip a workout or quit altogether. The only day you will repeat any exercise will be on workout day seven. That's your semi-rest day. When you get to that workout chapter, you'll see that I allow you to go back and pick any two buttocks exercises and any two abdominal exercises found in previous workouts. By day seven, you'll appreciate the freedom of choice. You'll look forward to the change of pace.

If any exercise program should not bore you, it's this one. However, if you are occasionally bored, so what? Working out is not equivalent to viewing a television show, where boredom would merit an immediate press on the remote control. Forget about keeping yourself amused. You can get that elsewhere. Think of your goal. It's to see results, right? You want a hard, sexy, healthy, energetic body. So if you're bored, bite the bullet. You'll be glad you did once you start seeing results.

WHAT ABOUT INJURY?

The beauty of this system is its built-in protection against injury. Self-preservation or natural instinct will prevent you from squeezing or flexing so hard that you will hurt yourself. A 20-year-old athlete and his 65-year-old grandmother can perform the same exercise—each exerting the maximum pressure possible, and neither will get hurt. If the actual force exerted were measured, the 20-year-old would naturally have exerted more pressure, but the 65-year-old would have exerted her maximum amount—so both will see results, and neither will have been injured.

HOW BIG WILL
YOUR MUSCLES GROW?

Perhaps this question is best answered by stating what will not happen. You will *not* look like Arnold Schwarzenegger or Miss Olympia. Your muscles will develop and combine into a tight, strong, dense symmetry. You'll have a body that resembles a lean athlete. Your muscles will be closer in size and shape to gymnasts, dancers, martial artists, swimmers, or all-around athletes.

Don't worry. You won't get too big. In order for muscles to grow beyond a natural size, you must lift progressively heavier and heavier weights. It has been my experience that most men and women do not wish to build bulky muscles. What they do want is tight, hard muscle that makes for a lean, athletic look. This workout was created to fill that need.

HOW DOES THIS PROGRAM COMPARE TO OTHER METHODS OF GETTING IN SHAPE?

Nautilus circuit training. The Nautilus circuit training method of bodybuilding is designed to exercise all nine body parts, and at the same time to stimulate the heart and lungs. It is, in effect, an aerobic workout using weights. The participant is asked to do one exercise on a given machine or station and to move quickly to the next machine or station. The entire body is worked each exercise session (each session takes about 20 to 30 minutes and more ambitious participants are encouraged to go around the circuit an additional one or two times). What is accomplished is great conditioning for the heart and lungs and some stimulation of the muscles. What is not accomplished is any total body shaping.

Aerobics. An aerobic exercise is one in which you get your pulse rate up to between 70 and 80 percent of its maximum capacity and keep it there for at least 20 minutes. (To figure out your maximum pulse rate, subtract your age from 220.) Aerobic exercises such as running, jumping rope, riding a bicycle, or swimming are excellent for strengthening heart and lungs. Marathon runners must have the leanest, strongest heart muscles in the world. I'm not making light of the importance of having excellently conditioned heart and lungs. We need them for good health and for breathing efficiency. But for some of us it's not enough to have a lean heart and strong lungs. We are vain creatures and we like to see our bodies in perfect form. Aerobic activities cannot accomplish this. The only highly developed body parts on runners are their calves. Swimmers have terrific latissimus dorsi development (the athletic "V"), and bike riders have great thighs. But what about the rest of their bodies? The point is that aerobics are great—in their place. But they can't replace a total-body workout. (See Chapter 9 for optional aerobic exercises *in addition* to this program.)

Ball Sports. Tennis, racquetball, squash, paddleball, golf, and, stretching the "ball" idea to include a puck, hockey—all these sports provide an aerobic workout (if done vigorously enough) and provide a workout for various body parts (especially the arms, upper back, and shoulders) but they do not provide a planned total-body reshaping. Only scientific working with the principles of bodybuilding can do that.

The martial arts. As mentioned before, those who are active in the martial arts achieve small, dense, perfectly formed muscles by combining isometric pressure and dynamic tension in their "Katas"—dancelike practice sessions where fighting movements are simulated in slow motion. But there is a catch. Martial artists invest a minimum of 10 hours a week in their workouts.

Regular bodybuilding. You can achieve a perfectly formed, symmetrical body by working with weights the traditional bodybuilding way (as described in *Now or Never*), but you would have to use progressively heavier weights and work a minimum of five hours a week. The muscles achieved would be at least slightly larger than those which will result from working with this 12-minute program—but a lot more time and equipment would be required.

WHO CAN USE THIS WORKOUT?

- Women (and men, too) who want to become tight and toned as opposed to muscle-bound.

- Anyone who does not have the time and/or the desire to go to a gym.

- People who travel a lot and need a portable workout that takes the minimum of time.

- Anyone who wishes to learn the basic bodybuilding movements and break in gently before joining a gym and working with heavier weights.

- Those who ordinarily work out in a gym but wish to take a layoff from the gym workout without losing what they have achieved in muscular development.

- People who, for medical reasons, cannot lift heavy weights (but check with your doctor).

- Anyone who has sustained an injury to a particular body part and does not want that part to get out of shape, or to risk reinjury to that body part (but consult your doctor regarding your condition before starting this program).

HOW LONG WILL IT TAKE TO SEE AND FEEL RESULTS?

You'll feel tighter, stronger, and more fit in one week. In *three weeks* you'll actually begin to *see* results. Not only will your entire body feel harder—but you will begin to *look* tighter and more toned. You'll notice a difference when you catch a glance of yourself in a mirror in the morning as you're getting dressed or when you observe your body when taking a bath or shower. In *three months* every part of your body will be more shapely. People will begin to notice. In *six months,* you won't have an ounce of unwanted fat anywhere! You'll be perfect. You'll love yourself. (Of course, you'll also have to follow the food guidelines in Chapters 11 and 12.)

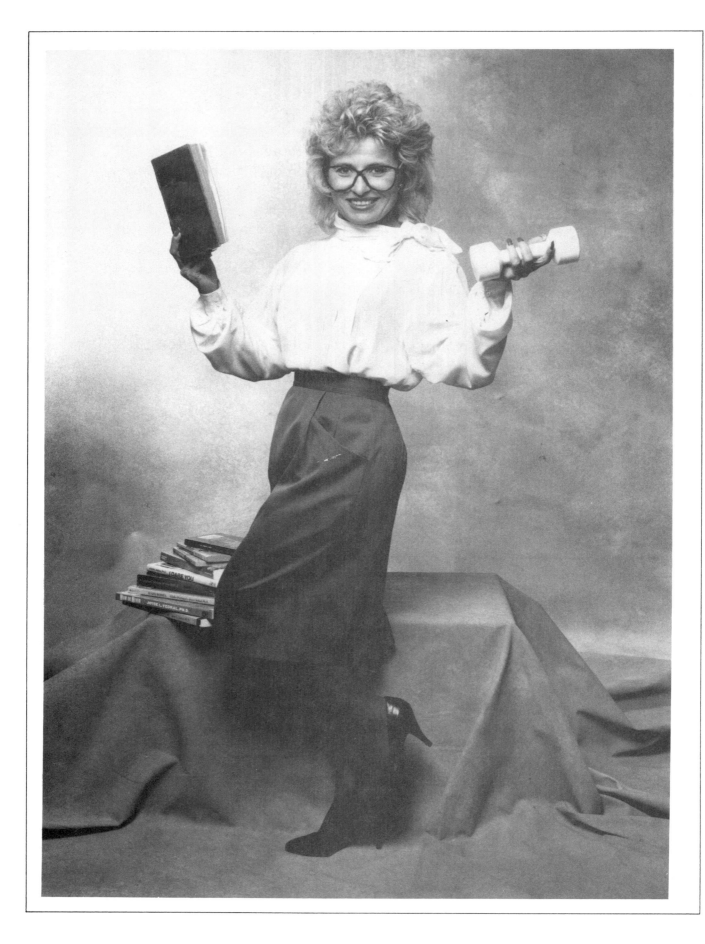

2

THE MIND, THE MOOD, AND THE MOVEMENT

It's all in your mind—and indeed it is. One day as you're getting dressed, you catch a glimpse of your body in the mirror, and you say to yourself, Bad news. Thank God so and so can't see me now. Two days later you again glance at your unclothed body, but this time you smile and say, Hmmm. Not so bad. All I have to do is get rid of this . . . and I'll look pretty good.

LEVELS OF CONSCIOUSNESS

Your level of consciousness is how you view the world at any given moment. It might be compared to looking at the world through rose-tinted glasses— or dark gray-tinted glasses. When you're in a low state of mind, you create negative thoughts and feelings to accompany that mood. On day one, you were probably feeling a bit down. Maybe you woke up to a cloudy day, were disturbed by a bad dream, were worrying about a difficult business situation, had had an argument with a loved one—or all four. But two days later, you wake up to the sunshine, after a great night's sleep and pleasant dreams—your business and personal problems resolved.

What does all this have to do with the *12-Minute Total-Body Workout?* Everything. When you start this program, you make a commitment to your body and to your mind—one that requires the devotion of 12 minutes per day, every day. At times you'll be tempted to skip a workout, not because you don't have the time or because you're too tired, but because you're "not in the mood." Once you realize that it's your level of consciousness that's stopping you from working out, and that you can control your level of consciousness, you'll no longer be the victim of what happens to be going on in your mind at a given moment.

Any bad mood can be lessened if, by an act of will, you begin to count your blessings (family, friends, health, security, peace of mind, luxuries, etc.). Once you start dwelling on the good things in your life, you'll realize that your life isn't as bad as you thought it was, and that things could be a lot worse than they are. No matter what's going on, it's not the situation alone that can hurt you, but the way you think about the situation.

Sometimes it's difficult to change your mood or raise your level of consciousness on command—even if you are fully aware of what's going on in your mind. When this happens, sheer logic can help you to take action even if your emotions are lagging behind.

IF YOU'RE TEMPTED TO SKIP A WORKOUT, THINK OF THIS

1. You're probably tempted to skip a workout because of your low level of consciousness.

2. Which will cause you regret later in the day? Working out or skipping a workout? Face it, if you do work out, there's no way you will regret it later. In fact, you will be happy and feel good about yourself when you think, I worked out this morning. But if you do skip a workout, you're sure to regret it later.

3. The investment of a mere 12 minutes a day will net you a tight, sensual body, better health, more energy, and a youthful appearance. You waste more time than that daydreaming, talking on the telephone, and certainly watching television.

MAINTAIN A
SENSE OF HUMOR

Take the pressure off yourself. You want to get into shape not so that you can win a beauty prize, but because you want to feel better about yourself and how you look. Stand in front of a full-length mirror. Take an "ugly stance." Push your stomach out, hunch your shoulders, bend your knees a little, and look as unshapely as possible. Now grin foolishly at yourself and say out loud, "Hi." If you're not laughing by now, shuffle across the room in that posture saying, "I look good." Imagine yourself doing this in front of the person you would most like to impress with your physical beauty or prowess. *So what!* Right? No matter what shape you're in, it isn't the end of the world. After all, what will it matter a hundred years from now that you had flabby thighs or a potbelly?

Humor increases endorphins, your body's natural opiates. If you can laugh at yourself, the chemicals released to your body will give you a "natural high" and you'll feel the pressure lifting. You'll find it much easier to do your daily exercises if you don't take yourself so seriously.

THE POWER
OF THE MIND

And while we are talking about moods, let's remember that the mind affects not only our moods, but our energy, our health, our eating habits, and even the shape of our bodies. Dr. Bernie S. Siegel, author of *Love, Medicine and Miracles,* says, "...the state of our mind has an immediate and direct effect on our state of body....By visualizing certain changes, we can help the body bring them about."[1] Dr. Siegel further points out that patients of his have been able to use their minds to direct chemotherapy to kill a cancerous tumor or to cut off the blood supply to a cancerous tumor, while ordering chemotherapy *not* to affect hair-growth cells (loss of hair usually occurs when chemotherapy is given, because hair-growth cells, like cancer cells, are rapid-growth cells).[2]

It is common knowledge that placebos have helped cure people of various ailments, even though these sugar pills in and of themselves have absolutely no medicinal value. But we now know that the mind is even capable of taking a medication that would ordinarily be harmful to the body and cause that drug to help the body.

I'm not telling you that in order to succeed in this workout you must practice using your mind as described in this chapter. However, I believe it is possible to speed up your metabolism by using your mind. Dr. Donald Wilson has experimented with patients who were able to do this by picturing a mental switch that turns the metabolism on and off. By turning this switch "on" every night before bedtime, patients were able to speed up their metabolism and burn additional calories during sleep to accelerate weight loss.[3] I have tried this mental exercise before bedtime, when I feel especially sluggish, and it seems to work. I can literally feel my body tingling and active during my sleep.

PRE-CONDITION YOURSELF TO CONTROL CONSUMPTION OF UNHEALTHY FOODS

Now on to the subject of food. Most people who indulge in high-calorie foods would have no problem with these foods if they didn't overdo it. For example, if you like ice-cream and you have one scoop a week, there will be no problem. But the fact is, you probably eat more than that. That's how you gain weight. In order to stop yourself from overeating your favorite unhealthy food treat, set a mental cut-off point by pre-conditioning your mind to alert you when you are about to indulge in the food. Using the ice-cream example, suppose you have achieved your weight goal and are now eating whatever you want once a week, on your free eating day, and you choose ice-cream. (See Chapter 11, "Making Friends with Food" for details on this program.) Tell yourself ahead of time, When I eat the ice-cream, I'm going to enjoy one large scoop. My body will rejoice in the treat, because it will be used to eating nutritious, healthy foods, and will welcome the change. But my body is a fine-tuned instrument now. It will not tolerate an excess of non-nutritious foods. If I eat more than one scoop, I'll begin to have a queasy feeling in my stomach. When I get ready to eat that second scoop, I'll get up, put the ice-cream back in the container, and walk away feeling great.

You can use this method to help you with any food item that tempts you to indulge. If you do this, you will not be merely hypnotizing yourself. You'll be helping your body to achieve what it really desires, because while your body can tolerate non-nutritious foods in limited quantities, it does not thrive on them. It's usually your mind, not your body, that causes you to overeat these foods, so why not use your mind to get things under control.

USING YOUR MIND TO HELP YOU WITH THIS WORKOUT

In order to be successful with this workout, it is crucial that you establish a strong mind-body connection, because this workout is based upon isometric and dynamic tension movements, which require mental cooperation. (See pages 23-24 for a full discussion of this subject.) It is absolutely necessary that you throw your mind into the body part you are working. This means total concentration on what you are doing.

As I've already noted, this workout requires that you exercise three body parts each day (except for Sundays when you exercise only two body parts). Each day, before you begin your workout, think about the body parts you will be exercising. For example, on Monday you will work on chest, shoulders, and triceps, so on that day, stand before the mirror and locate these body parts (see anatomy photo if you are unfamiliar with their exact location) and focus your mental energy on them in preparation for the workout. Picture these specific body parts being energized and developed even before you make the first move with the dumbbells. It only takes a second, but it will greatly increase your results. Then, when you begin your first exercise, which is a chest exercise, mentally isolate your chest from all other body parts and give total concentration to that body part. As you pick up the dumbbells, you will move them with one thing in mind and one thing only: chest development. Your entire body is engaged in a dance that is featuring chest. You will do this for each and every body part each time you exercise. In time, you will do this automatically, but in the beginning you'll continually have to call your mind back to the body part you are working.

VISUALIZE CHANGE AS YOU EXERCISE EACH BODY PART

It is not enough to focus on the body part as you exercise. You must also visualize that muscle getting harder and more shapely. Picture the ideal shape you have in mind for that muscle, and as you move the dumbbells, tell your muscle to get into that shape. This program will not allow your muscles to become overly large, so don't waste your time picturing gargantuan muscles. Imagine small, perfectly formed muscles taking shape, and spongy, unsightly fat being worn away as you work.

VISUALIZE YOUR NEW BODY

Take an "anatomy photo" of yourself, something like the one I took on pages 30-31. Make two copies of each picture, front and back. Label one set just as I did, and place it in a private but convenient place. You'll use these later to see how your body has changed after a few months. Now take the other set and, using a thin-line felt pen, "correct" the picture. If your buttocks are too low, raise them with the pen. If your stomach is jutting out, cut off the excess with the pen. If your thighs are too large, slim them down with the pen—and so on. Draw larger biceps and calves if necessary and reshape your shoulders. Do whatever you have to do to give yourself the perfect body. The "corrected" picture is your goal. Instruct your body to take the "corrected" form. Give it a time span in which to achieve the result—something comfortable. Ask yourself how long it should take. You'll sense a realistic answer (somewhere between two and six months). Periodically look at the original and "corrected" picture and compare both against what you see in the mirror. Each time you do this, tell yourself (your mind tells your body): Work toward that goal. Get into that shape. The mind is somewhat like a homing torpedo. When given a goal, it will strive to achieve that goal—and will zigzag its way around obstacles in order to achieve it. But you have to cooperate by periodically repeating the instructions.

THE DANCE OF THE
MIND AND THE MOVEMENT

As you exercise, perform each movement with your mind. Relax as you work, even though you will be tensing your muscles continually. Let yourself become mesmerized in the rhythm of the movement and the total concentration of your mind as you are free of every interfering thought. Your exercise session will provide an interlude—a brief vacation from life.

POSITIVE PSYCHOLOGICAL BENEFITS OF THIS PROGRAM

Unlike other fitness programs, the *12-Minute Total-Body Workout* provides closure: You are doing something to help your body every single day. This daily effort helps you to feel in control, and what starts out as a feeling of control of what happens to your body ends up in a feeling that you are in control of your life.

Nathaniel Branden, the renowned psychologist, says that self-esteem is a man's reputation with himself. Doing your daily 12-minute routine helps to build self-esteem, because you aim at—and achieve—a goal every day, and thus build a good reputation with yourself. This small daily achievement tells you, in a subtle way, that you're reliable and responsible, and indicates to you that you can also accomplish much more difficult goals.

In addition, working with this program causes your body language to change. Where you once walked with poor posture, you now find yourself throwing your shoulders back, tightening your abdominal muscles, and walking with an in-control stride. Before, your body language was saying, I'm getting older. I'm tired, I'm not proud of my appearance, I feel defeated. Now, your body language says, I'm energetic, I feel good about myself. I can make things happen.

Whenever you happen to touch your own body, you'll notice that you no longer feel soft and flaccid, but tight and toned. Because of the nature of the workout (constant dynamic tension and isometric pressure), you'll find that your muscles are automatically flexed most of the time. This will send you a message: I'm strong. I'm healthy. I'm sensual. Others will also get the message.

HOW TO USE YOUR MIND TO GET THE MAXIMUM BENEFIT FROM THIS WORKOUT

• Read the entire book before you start and absorb the logic of the program.

• Realize that you have the power to change your life. You've achieved other goals, haven't you?

- Forgive yourself for being in the shape you are in.

- Maintain a sense of humor. Don't take yourself so seriously; after all, what will it really matter a hundred years from now?

- Use the power of your mind to control your diet and to reshape your body.

- Concentrate on the body part you are exercising and that body part only.

- Visualize your ideal body and remind your body to achieve that goal.

- Understand that just as the mind affects the body, the body affects the mind. An in-shape body helps you to be happy and positive about your life.

- Watch for changes in your body language after one month on this program.

- Be alert to psychological carry-over after two weeks on this program.

NOTES

[1] Bernie S. Siegel, M.D., *Love, Medicine and Miracles* (New York: Harper & Row, 1986), p. 69.

[2] Ibid., pp. 131–135, 152–155.

[3] Donald M. Wilson, M.D., *Total Mind Power* (New York: Berkley Books Inc., 1978), pp. 81–91.

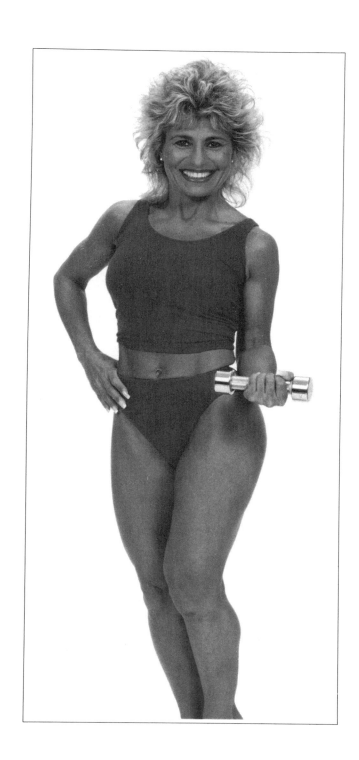

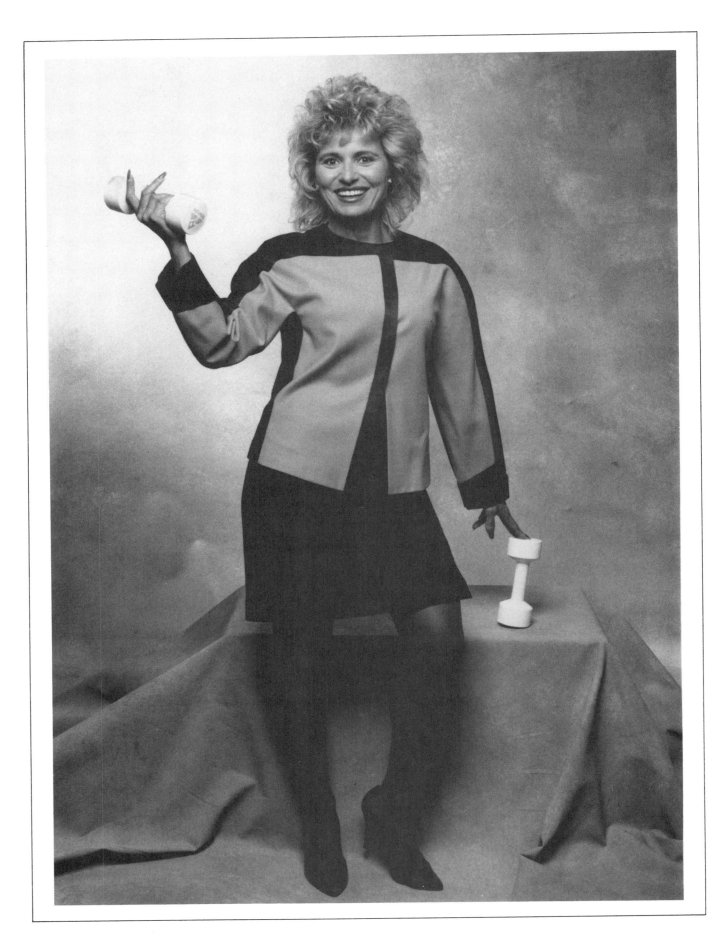

3

A Pair of Three-Pound Dumbbells and You're in Business

The easiest part of this workout is buying your equipment. The three-pound dumbbells can be purchased in any sporting goods store, or you can order them from me.[1] The more difficult part is understanding exactly what you have to do with those dumbbells and why you have to do it, but by the time you finish reading this chapter, you'll know everything you need to know—and a lifetime of fitness will have begun.

In order to make your workout simple, you should familiarize yourself with the following exercise terms. These terms will be used again and again in your daily routine.

Exercise Terminology

Exercise. The particular movement you execute in order to develop or challenge a specific muscle. For example, the dumbbell curl is a biceps exercise.

Repetition, or rep. One complete movement of an exercise from start to midpoint and back to start again.

Set. A number of repetitions performed in sequence without stopping. In this program, you will be performing 10 repetitions for each set of each exercise, and three total sets of each exercise. More about that later.

Rest. In this workout, a 5-to-10-second pause between sets. The rest enables you to gather strength for your next set.

Routine. All of the exercises performed for a particular body part on a given day. For example, in this workout, your Monday chest routine consists of two exercises: a flat isometric dumbbell press and an incline isometric dumbbell flye.

Workout. The total of all exercises performed on a given day. For example, in this program, your Monday workout will consist of your entire chest, shoulder, and triceps routines. You will have performed two exercises for each of these body parts, and you will have performed three sets of 10 repetitions each for every exercise. More about this later.

MUSCLES: GROWTH, SHAPE, AND MOVEMENT

Your skeleton is the body's frame or underpinning structure. Your internal organs such as heart, lungs, intestines, etc. function to keep your body alive. Your blood flows throughout your body supplying nourishment for your heart, lungs, etc., and your skin covers your entire body. But it is muscles that determine your shape.

I say to myself, How silly, when I hear a woman say, "I don't want to get muscles." Doesn't she know that she already *has* muscles? It's the muscles under her skin and that are attached to her bones that give her body whatever shape and tone she has—and that shape depends on how well formed those muscles are, and how much fat is covering those muscles.

You do need muscles. In fact, if you're not careful, your muscles will atrophy and become flaccid. You'll look and feel soft and spongy, or fat. The goal of this workout is to take the muscles you already have and make them firm, tight, tense, and perfectly formed and to put small shapely muscles where they are not visible because, due to lack of challenge, they have shrunk to microscopic size.

Don't be afraid of muscles. Even men tell me they don't want to get big muscles. What you'll get with this program is quality muscle—not quantity.

There are three aspects to muscles that must be understood in order to appreciate this program fully. They are muscle quality, muscle action, and muscle description.

MUSCLE QUALITY TERMS

Density. The quality of hardness in a muscle. The main feature of this program is its ability to produce muscle density. Because of the continual pressure being exerted on the working muscle, the muscle is condensed and solidified first. Then and only then does it grow.

Definition. The condition of a muscle when it is relatively free of surrounding fat. For example, after working with this program for a few months, your abdominal muscles will become well defined because, as you develop your muscles and follow good eating habits, your abdominals will be relatively free of the fat that used to surround and hence obscure them.

MUSCLE ACTION TERMS

Squeezing, or Flexing. To squeeze or flex a muscle is to exert maximum pressure on a working muscle as it moves into a contracted position. For example, when performing the dumbbell curl, you squeeze or flex the muscle as hard as possible as you curl the dumbbell upward toward your shoulders. In this workout, I prefer the term *squeeze* to *flex*, because flex has taken on the connotation of squeezing just on the high or midpoint of the exercise. In this workout, you continually squeeze the muscle.

Isometric pressure. The force exerted on the muscle as it is being squeezed, flexed, or shortened, as opposed to dynamic tension (below). For example, isometric pressure is applied to your biceps muscle when you are performing a biceps curl, as you curl your arm upward into the fist-to-shoulder position.

Dynamic tension. The force exerted on the muscle as it is being elongated, extended, or stretched. For example, dynamic tension is applied to your biceps muscle when you are performing a biceps curl, as you extend your arm downward.

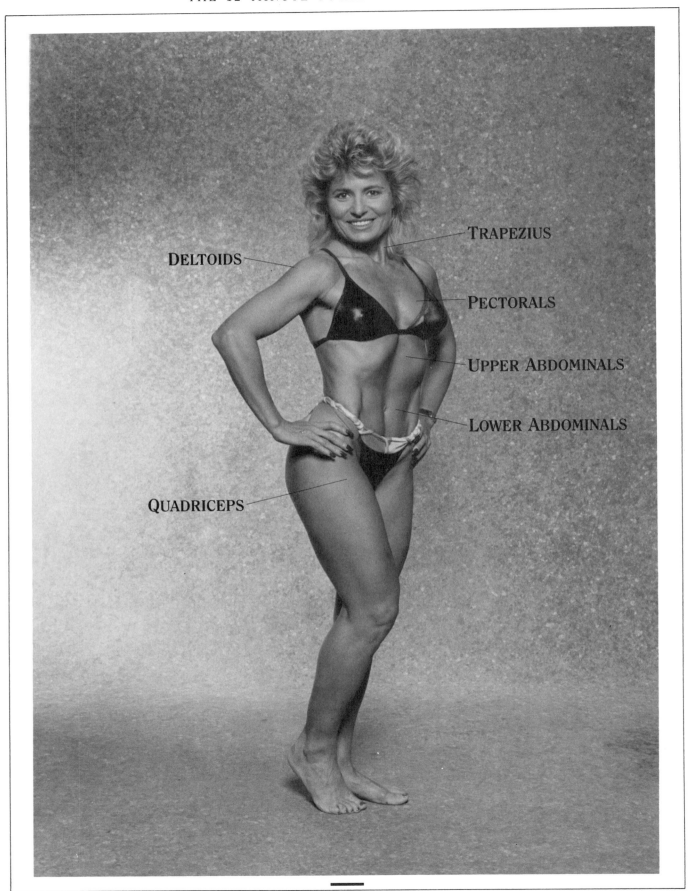

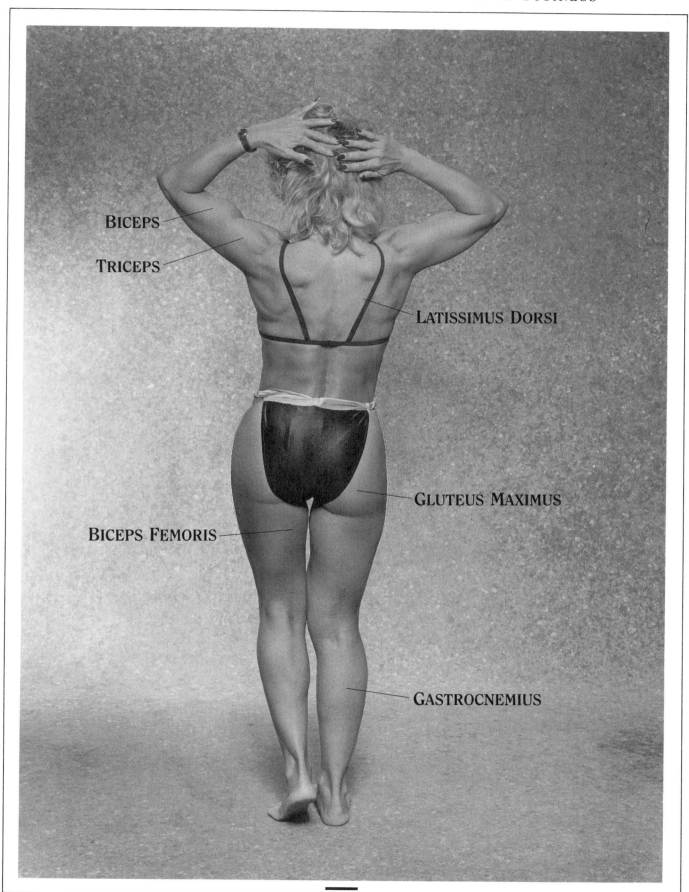

MUSCLE DESCRIPTION

In order to gain the maximum results from this exercise program, it is crucial that you understand at all times exactly what your goal is as you work each muscle. In order to do this, you should know a little bit about each muscle and how the particular exercises in this program challenge these muscles. This program covers all nine body parts or muscle groups. They are, in the order in which they appear in the workout: chest, shoulders, triceps, thighs, buttocks, abdominals, back, biceps, and calves. Refer to the anatomy photographs on pages 30-31 as you read these descriptions.

Chest. The muscles located just under your breasts are fanlike in shape and are called pectorals. They work to move your arms. They consist of two muscle groups, upper and medial. This workout provides a full exercise program for all aspects of your pectoral muscles. On Monday you will do the flat isometric dumbbell press, which works your entire pectoral area, and the incline isometric dumbbell flye, which specifically challenges your upper pectoral area. On Thursday, your second chest workout day, you will do a standing isometric dumbbell crossover, which develops the inner pectoral muscle and helps to produce the well-defined look of cleavage or separation, and the seated isometric chest squeeze, which challenges the entire pectoral muscle and again specifically helps to develop the inner area of that muscle to produce a separated, defined look.

Shoulders. These muscles are technically called deltoids. They are three-headed muscles that help to raise the arms. This workout helps to develop the three heads: *front,* or *anterior,* muscles, which work as you move your arms in a forward direction; *side,* or *medial,* muscles, which help to move your arms out to the sides; and *rear,* or *posterior,* muscles, which work to move your arms in a backwards direction. On Monday you will do a front isometric lateral raise, which works the anterior deltoid muscle, and a pee-wee rear lateral raise, which works the posterior deltoid muscle. On Thursday, your second shoulder workout day, you will do a standing isometric side lateral raise, which works your medial deltoid muscles, and a bent-over isometric lateral raise, which works your posterior and medial deltoid muscles.

Triceps. The triceps is a three-headed muscle that consists of an *inner, outer,* and *medial* head. All three heads of the muscle are attached to the shoulder blade. Their job is to extend the forearm and arm, and to help pull back the arm once it is extended. It is the triceps muscle that causes most women grief after the late twenties, since it is probably the most neglected muscle on the human body. It is the one that, if not exercised, waves like a flag when the arm is extended. On Monday you will do a double-arm isometric kickback, which works to develop the entire triceps muscle, especially the outer head, and an isometric overhead extension, which again works the entire triceps muscle, but especially stresses the inner and medial heads of that muscle. On Thursday, your second triceps workout day, you will do a kneeling isometric dumbbell pulldown, which exercises the entire triceps muscle, especially the inner head, and a standing isometric dumbbell pushdown, which exercises the entire triceps muscle, especially the outer head.

Thighs. The front thigh is called the *quadriceps* muscle because it consists of four muscles that travel along the front thigh and end in the kneecap. These muscles work to extend the leg from a bent position. The back thigh or *biceps femoris*—hamstrings—are made up of three muscles that are located on the back outside of the thigh and insert through the inside of the knee. These muscles work together to rotate the leg, extend the hips, and flex the knee. On Tuesday you will do a fingertip isometric squat, which exercises your complete quadriceps muscle as well as your buttocks, and a dumbbell isometric lunge, which exercises your quadriceps muscle along with your hips and buttocks. On Friday, your second weekly thigh workout, you will do a seated isometric leg extension, which exercises your quadriceps muscle, and a lying isometric leg curl, which exercises your biceps femoris muscle.

Buttocks. The buttock muscle is called the *gluteus maximus* because it is the largest muscle in the body. It runs from the hipbone to the tailbone, and works to extend and rotate the thigh. All four buttocks exercises work the entire gluteus maximus muscle. On Tuesday you will do the dumbbell isometric standing squeeze and the kneeling isometric angled leg lift. On Friday, your second weekly buttocks workout day, you will do the seated isometric scissor and the kneeling isometric feather kick-up. On Sunday, your third weekly buttocks exercise day, you will select any two of the four buttocks exercises. It doesn't matter which ones.

Abdominals. Although technically the abdominal muscle (*rectus abdominis*) is a single long, slender muscle that rises from the ribs near the breastbone and runs vertically along the abdominal wall, it is considered to be plural for several reasons. First, it is a segmented muscle, hence the term *abs*. Second, for workout purposes, the abdominal area is divided into two parts, *upper* and *lower*. This is due to the fact that it is impossible to contract both upper and lower areas of the abdominal muscles fully at the same time. The abdominal muscles work to pull the torso toward the lower body, and are used in some way in almost every exercise. In your Tuesday workout, you will do a dumbbell isometric sit-up, which challenges your upper abdominal area, and a dumbbell isometric leg-raise, which challenges your lower abdominal area. In your Friday workout, your second weekly abdominal workout, you will do a seated isometric leg-in, which exercises your lower abdominal area, and an isometric crunch, which exercises your upper abdominal area. On Sunday, your third weekly abdominal exercise day, you will select any of the above abdominal exercises. It is a good idea to choose one upper and one lower abdominal exercise.

Back. The most important back muscles are the *latissimus dorsi,* or "lats," because they provide the "V" shape to the back when properly developed. The other back muscles that will concern us are the *trapezius* and the upper back muscles. The latissimus dorsi, or "lats," rise along the spinal column from the middle of the back to the tailbone. The "lats" are used to help pull the shoulder back and the arm toward the body. The two large trapezius muscles run on either side of the spine from the back of the neck to the middle of the back. They work to support the head and shoulders. Some fitness experts consider the trapezius muscles to be shoulder muscles, since they can be seen between the neck and shoulder area, from a front view, when well developed. The upper back muscles consist of many muscles such as the *rhomboideus major and minor, teres major and minor,* etc. These muscles work to pull and rotate the arm and shoulder. On Wednesday you will do seated isometric back laterals, which work your upper back and trapezius muscles, and standing isometric leaning pulls, which exercise your latissimus dorsi and upper back muscles. On Saturday, your second weekly back workout, you will do isometric bent dumbbell rows, which exercise the latissimus dorsi and trapezius muscles, and isometric lat pulldowns, which challenge your latissimus dorsi muscles.

Biceps. The biceps is a two-headed muscle (hence the term *biceps* as opposed to *bicep*). The muscle originates in the shoulder blade and ends in the forearm. Although the muscle has two heads, unless one is a champion bodybuilder and has developed the muscle to the extreme of having two heads visible, it appears to be a single muscle that shows up as a curve about halfway down the upper arm. The biceps works to bend or flex the arm at the elbow. Each biceps exercise challenges the entire biceps muscle. On Wednesday you will do seated alternating isometric dumbbell curls and leaning isometric concentration curls. On Saturday, your second weekly biceps workout, you will do isometric preacher dumbbell curls and standing isometric simultaneous dumbbell curls.

Calves. The calf muscles are comprised of the *gastrocnemius* and the *soleus* muscles. The gastrocnemius is divided into two parts, which connect in the middle of the lower leg and tie in with the Achilles tendon. The section where the two heads of the muscle form the tie constitutes the bulge of the calf muscle. The job of the gastrocnemius muscle is to flex the knee and foot downward. The soleus muscle is located underneath the gastrocnemius muscle. It assists the gastrocnemius in flexing the foot downward. Each calf exercise challenges both gastrocnemius and soleus muscles. Because the calf muscles are easily developed, and because they receive natural stimulation in walking and running, only one calf exercise per workout day is necessary. On Wednesday you will do a seated isometric calf raise, and on Saturday you will do a standing one-leg isometric dumbbell calf raise.

LOGIC OF
EXERCISE GROUPINGS

You may wonder why I selected chest, shoulders, and triceps to be exercised together on a given day and thighs, buttocks, and abdominals on another day, and so on. Many years of bodybuilding expertise have proven that certain body parts are best worked with certain other body parts.

Chest, Shoulders, and Triceps. Chest and shoulders are closely linked in the work they do. Physiologically, they tie into one another. By linking them, you are able to exercise those muscle groups thoroughly and give them the greatest possible challenge. The biceps is a smaller muscle than your pectoral or deltoid (chest or shoulder) muscles. It is included not only to balance out the workout but to isolate it from the triceps muscle (the other arm muscle) so that your arm won't become overly exhausted and miss the maximum benefit of the workout. This is a very demanding exercise program. (Using isometric pressure and dynamic tension is lots of work, as you will see.)

Thighs, buttocks, abdominals. The front and back thigh muscles are linked to the buttocks muscles, and so, in order to provide a complete challenge to these muscle groups, they are exercised on the same day. It is the abdominal muscles that provide the center of your strength. They come into play with nearly every exercise you do. They can be exercised conveniently on any workout day, and since you must work them three times a week, and I like to leave a day between workouts for any given body part, your first workout cannot be later in the week than Tuesday.

Back, biceps, calves. The remaining muscle groups—back, biceps, and calves—are completely unrelated to each other, and can be exercised on the same day without exhausting one another.

Buttocks and abdominals. These two muscle groups are often exercised together on an additional exercise day, because they must be worked more often than most other muscles. They are grouped together on day seven strictly for convenience—to fit them into the workout.

WHEN AND WHERE SHOULD YOU WORK OUT?

The beauty of this program is its flexibility. You can completely cater to your own needs. If you know you're the type of person who hates to lift a finger after a hard day's work—or if you feel you would dread even this short 12-minute routine all day, then do it as soon as you jump out of bed in the morning. If, on the other hand, you are well disciplined and know that you would use the routine to relieve the tension of a hard day's work, do it in the evenings. You can even work out during your lunch break.

You can work out at home, in your office, at a friend's home, in a motel—anywhere. I don't suggest you work out while watching television, however. You'll need total concentration in order to get the maximum results.

STRETCHING

All you have to do is loosen up a bit before you start your workout. Most people invent a few natural stretches before beginning a workout.

Here's an example of a natural stretching cycle that would take about a minute: Rotate your head a few times in each direction, then your trunk. Touch your toes a few times without bending your knees, right fingers to left toes, left fingers to right toes. Then lie on the floor and, with your legs apart, sit up, lean over, and without bending your knees, try to touch your head first to your left knee and then to your right knee. Stand up, shake out your arms and then each leg. You're ready to go.

YOUR DAILY ROUTINE

Do three sets of 10 repetitions for each exercise. (The only exceptions are buttocks and abdominals, in which case you can do as many as 25 repetitions once you've become accustomed to the workout, but this is optional.)

Rest 5-to-10 seconds between sets. Reminders are given at the beginning of each workout day.

BREAKING IN GENTLY

In most fitness programs, breaking in gently means beginning with a few exercises and gradually adding more exercises until the complete program is presented. This workout is different. You will start out by doing the full program immediately. But you will not exert the full force of isometric pressure and dynamic tension the first week.

For the first week of your workout, don't use any isometric pressure or dynamic tension. Just go through the motions of each exercise in order to learn the form. Because you're not using any pressure, the workout will take you about half the time, say, six minutes a day. You'll be tempted to swing the dumbbells because you're not using pressure, but instead, go rather slowly and concentrate on form.

For the second week I want you to exert some pressure, but not a lot. Think of yourself as exerting one-half of the pressure you will exert next week, at which time you'll exert the full force of your energy.

By week three, you're ready to give it everything you have. Exert the full force of isometric tension and dynamic tension. Your body will literally tingle.

As time goes by, you'll find yourself getting stronger and stronger, and you'll notice that you're able to exert even more force as you squeeze your muscles while doing the exercises. In a few months' time, your squeezing power will have doubled or tripled as your muscles become hard, strong, and well formed.

Please don't be impatient and try to exert the full force the first week. You'll lose the advantage of getting the feel of the program, and of sensing the capacity of your muscles to increase their power gradually.

ESTABLISHING A ROUTINE

It's important to set up a daily routine and to stick with it. For example, if you decide to work out in the morning, try to incorporate that 12-minute workout into your daily routine just as you allow time for brushing your teeth or taking a shower. Make it your business not to skip a workout, the same way you wouldn't skip brushing your teeth or showering. It is especially important not to skip workouts for the first month or two, because you are setting up a pattern that, when established, will give you a lifetime of fitness.

MAKING UP A WORKOUT

After this workout has become a normal part of your life, you may find yourself skipping a workout from time to time because of emergencies. If you skip a 12-minute total-body workout one day, you can make it up the next day by working out both in the morning and in the evening. For example, suppose you skip your Monday workout. On Tuesday morning, instead of doing your Tuesday workout, do your Monday workout. Then Tuesday evening, do your regular Tuesday workout. On Wednesday morning, you'll be back on course. Your body will behave as if you had worked out on Monday, as you always do. If you skip two days, you can perform double workouts two days in a row. For example, if you didn't work out Monday or Tuesday, you can do Monday's workout on Wednesday morning, and Tuesday's workout on Wednesday evening. Then you can do Wednesday's workout Thursday morning and Thursday's workout Thursday night. On Friday you'll be back on course. It isn't a good idea to get into the habit of missing more than one day of working out. One of the most important benefits of this program is its daily stimulation of your body.

If you skip one or two days' workout, and you don't feel like making it up, that's okay. Just forgive yourself and make up your mind to be more diligent. I don't want this program to become a burden to you. It should be a delightful experience, not an albatross around your neck. Make up the workout only if you know that doing so will put you in a better frame of mind and will make you feel good about yourself. The world won't end if you skip a workout or two once in a while, once the routine has been established as a normal part of your daily life.

NOTES

[1] To order my special cast-iron dumbbells, send a check or money order for $12.00 to: Joyce Vedral, P.O.B. A433, Wantagh, NY 11793-0433. You will pay shipping charges upon receipt.
For chrome dumbbells call Weider Health and Fitness, 1-800-423-5590 or 818-884-6800.

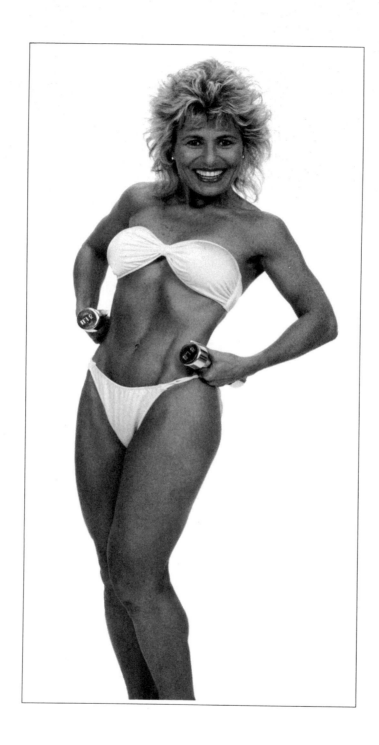

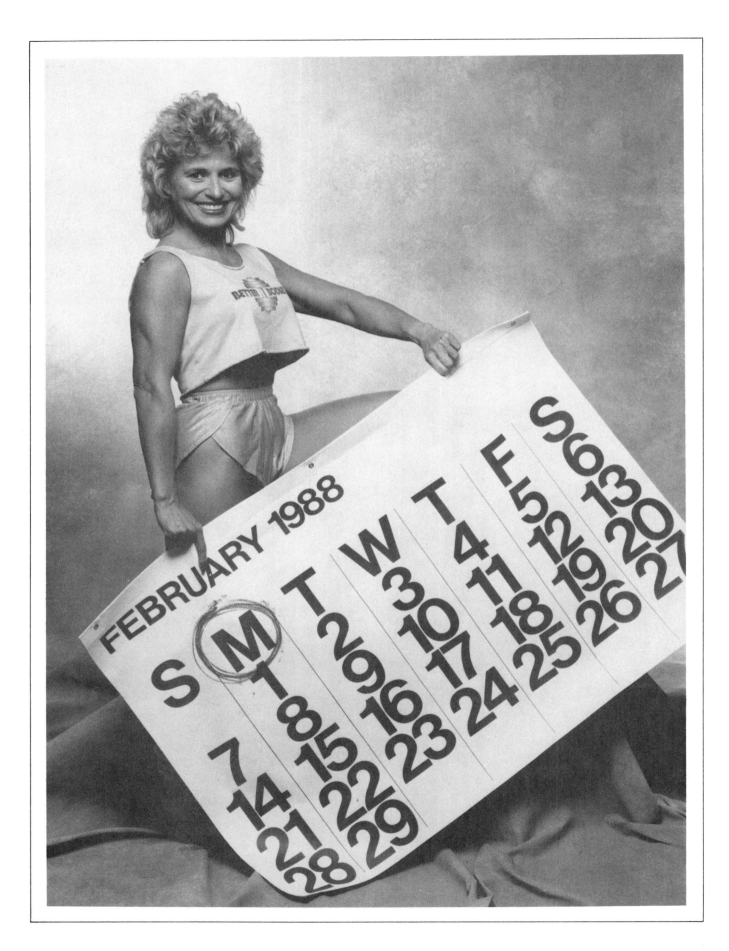

4

THE 12-MINUTE MONDAY WORKOUT

Today you're going to exercise three body parts: chest, shoulders, and triceps. You will do two exercises for each of them. The exercises are commonly referred to in shortened nickname form. (Nicknames for each exercise are given in quotes in parentheses. As you learn your exercises, memorize their nicknames rather than their longer forms. The term *ID* means "isometric-dynamic tension." It is used throughout this workout for the sake of brevity.

CHEST:	Flat ID dumbbell presses ("presses")
	Incline ID dumbbell flyes ("flyes")
SHOULDERS:	Front ID lateral raises ("front raises")
	Pee-wee ID rear lateral raises ("pee-wee laterals")
TRICEPS:	Double-arm ID kickbacks ("kickbacks")
	Double-arm ID overhead extensions ("extensions")
SETS AND REPETITIONS:	Do three sets of 10 repetitions each.
REST:	5-to-10 seconds between sets. (The same rest interval applied throughout the workout)
EQUIPMENT:	A pair of three-pound dumbbells
	A chair (any kitchen or desk chair will do)

FLAT ID DUMBBELL PRESSES— CHEST EXERCISE #1
("PRESSES")

Develops: Chest (breast) or pectoral muscles.

READY

Place your shoulders on the seat of a chair, with your feet together. Raise yourself onto the balls of your feet. Your back should be slightly arched.

SET

Hold a dumbbell in each hand, palms upward. The end of each dumbbell should touch your outer, upper breast area.

GO

Squeezing your pectoral muscles as hard as possible, as you apply isometric pressure, move the dumbbells upward until your arms are fully extended. Without resting, and applying the full force of dynamic tension, return to start position. Without resting, repeat the movement until you have finished your set. Complete your final two sets and immediately move to the next exercise.

ATTENTION

Don't hold your breath. Continually apply the force of isometric pressure and dynamic tension. Keep your mind on your pectoral muscles throughout the movement. You will be asked, time and again throughout the seven days of this workout, to apply isometric pressure and dynamic tension. To make things simple, however, all you have to do is to remember to squeeze, squeeze, squeeze—whenever you are in motion. You may do this exercise at the edge of your bed or on a flat exercise bench.

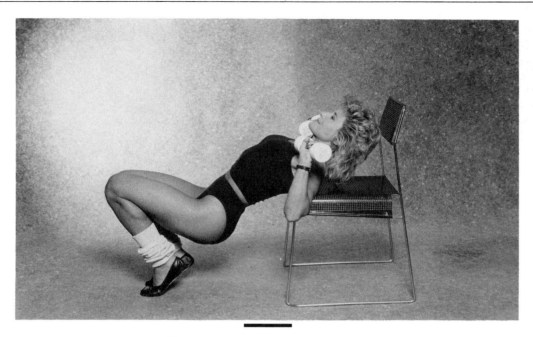

FLAT ID DUMBBELL PRESS
START

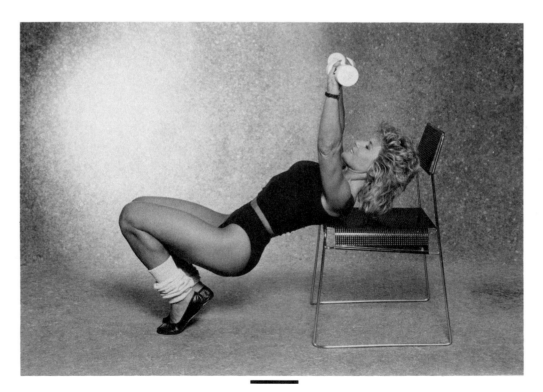

FLAT ID DUMBBELL PRESS
FINISH

INCLINE ID DUMBBELL FLYES–
CHEST EXERCISE #2
("FLYES")

Develops: Upper pectoral muscle, entire pectoral area.

READY

Sit in a chair, holding a three-pound dumbbell in each hand.

SET

Tip the chair back to an incline by leaning back and rising up on the balls of your feet. Don't worry—you won't fall; you can control the chair's tilt by lowering and raising your heels. Hold the dumbbells, palms facing inward, and extend your arms straight up. Your elbows should be slightly bent. Let the dumbbells touch each other above the center of your chest area.

GO

Using dynamic tension, extend your arms outward and downward in a semicircle until you feel a full stretch in your chest. Applying isometric pressure, return to start. Without resting, repeat the movement until you have finished your set. Complete your final two sets and immediately move to the next exercise.

ATTENTION

You will feel some pressure in your back and rear shoulder areas, but if you rivet your mind on your pectoral muscles, you will force them to do most of the work. You may do this exercise flat, at the edge of your bed or on an exercise bench.

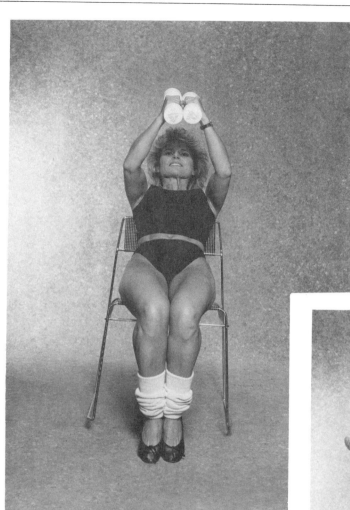

INCLINE ID DUMBBELL FLYE
START

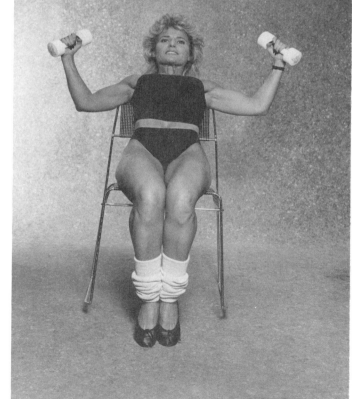

INCLINE ID DUMBBELL FLYE
FINISH

FRONT ID LATERAL RAISES– SHOULDER EXERCISE #1
("FRONT RAISES")

Develops: Front deltoid (shoulder) muscle.

READY

Stand with your feet shoulder-width apart, holding a dumbbell in each hand.

SET

Hold the dumbbells with your palms facing inward so that their ends touch your mid-thigh area. Your arms should be fully extended downward. Look straight ahead—into a mirror if possible.

GO

Squeezing your shoulders as hard as you can and applying isometric pressure, raise both dumbbells until they reach shoulder level. Applying the full power of dynamic tension, return to start position. Keep your elbows locked throughout the movement. Without resting, repeat the movement until you have finished your set. Complete your final two sets and immediately move on to the next exercise.

ATTENTION

In order to help yourself maintain the proper stiff-arm position throughout the exercise, think of yourself as Frankenstein's monster as you work. You will feel your triceps and lats working along with your front deltoids, but mentally focus all the attention on your front shoulders. This will help to get the maximum results for that area. You may also do this exercise by alternating arms.

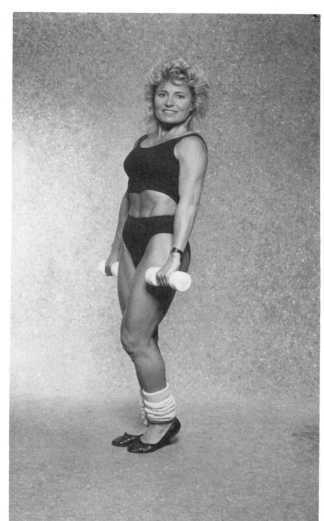

FRONT ID LATERAL RAISE
START

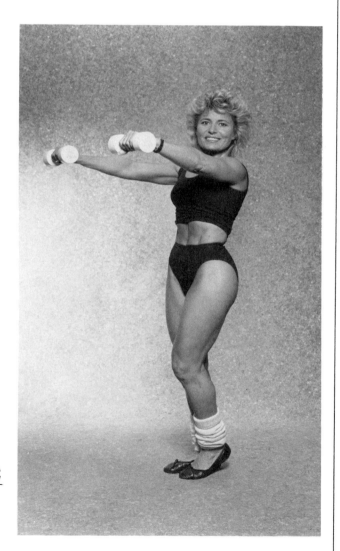

FRONT ID LATERAL RAISE
FINISH

PEE-WEE ID REAR LATERAL RAISES– SHOULDER EXERCISE #2
("PEE-WEE LATERALS")

Develops: Rear and medial deltoid (shoulder) muscles.

READY

Stand with your feet together, holding a dumbbell in each hand.

SET

Bending at the knees, thrust your hips forward and hold the dumbbells behind you, with palms facing inward and dumbbells touching each other. (The dumbbells will be grazing your lower buttocks area.)

GO

Squeezing your rear shoulder area as hard as possible, and applying isometric pressure, extend the dumbbells outward and upward in an arcing movement. Lead with your inward-bent, locked outer wrists and your elbows. Continue the movement until the dumbbells reach shoulder height and nearly touch each other. Applying dynamic tension, return to start and repeat the movement until you have finished your set. Complete your final two sets and immediately move to the next exercise.

ATTENTION

Maintain your hip-forward position throughout the movement. Continually use isometric pressure and dynamic tension. Focus your mind on the muscles you are exercising, your rear deltoids.

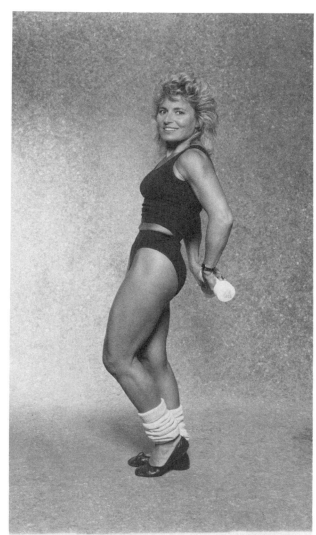

PEE-WEE ID REAR LATERAL RAISE
START

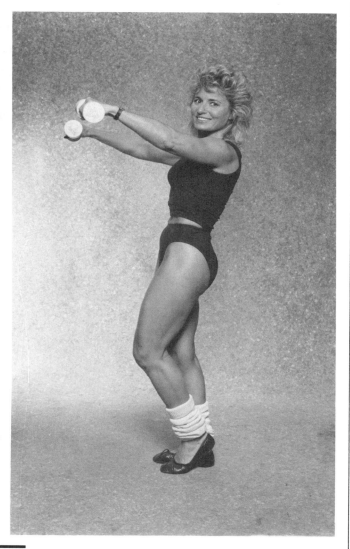

PEE-WEE ID REAR LATERAL RAISE
FINISH

DOUBLE-ARM ID KICKBACKS—TRICEPS EXERCISE #1
("KICKBACKS")

Develops: The entire triceps area, especially the
outer head of the muscle.

READY

Stand, with your feet together, bending at the waist and the knees, and holding a dumbbell in each hand, palms facing inward.

SET

Bend your elbows until the dumbbells are held in line with your chest (breast) area.

GO

Squeeze your triceps area as hard as possible, alying isometric pressure, move (or "kick") the dumbbells back behind you until your arms are fully extended and your elbows locked. Applying dynamic tension, return to start and repeat the movement until you have finished your set. Complete your final two sets and immediately move to the next exercise.

ATTENTION

The exercise may seem awkward at first, but you will soon gain a feel for it and you'll love it. Remember to keep the pressure and tension on throughout the exercise. You may feel your biceps working as well because the biceps works in opposition to your triceps—but keep your mind riveted on your triceps muscle. You may do this exercise one arm at a time by performing 10 repetitions for one arm, then switching to the other arm, and so on, until you have completed all three sets.

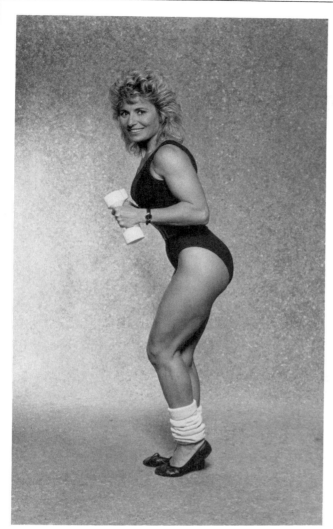

DOUBLE-ARM ID KICKBACK
START

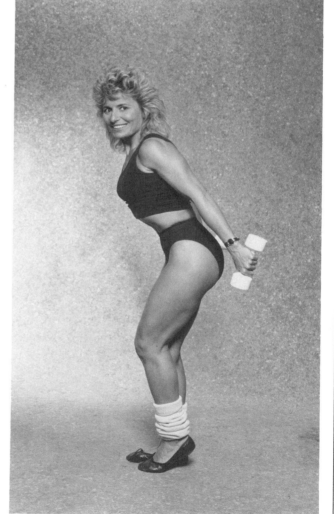

DOUBLE ARM ID KICKBACK
FINISH

DOUBLE-ARM ID OVERHEAD EXTENSIONS—TRICEPS EXERCISE #2

("EXTENSIONS")

Develops: The entire triceps area—especially the inner and middle heads of the muscle.

READY

Stand with feet together, holding one dumbbell with both hands.

SET

Raise the dumbbell above your head, holding it in both hands between your crossed fingers and thumbs, palms facing upward. Extend your arms straight up and pin your biceps to your ears.

GO

Using dynamic tension, lower the dumbbell behind your head. Continue lowering until the dumbbell touches the back of your neck. Applying isometric pressure, return to the start position and repeat the movement until you have finished your set. Complete your final two sets.

ATTENTION

You may perform this exercise one arm at a time. Do 10 repetitions for one arm, then switch to the other arm, and so on, until you have completed all three sets for each arm.

REMINDER

Isometric pressure is applied on the flexing part and dynamic tension is applied on the stretching part of this exercise—and all other exercises in this program, for that matter. The crucial thing to remember is, there is no point to any exercise during which you are relaxing. You must continually apply pressure—on both the up and down movement of each exercise.

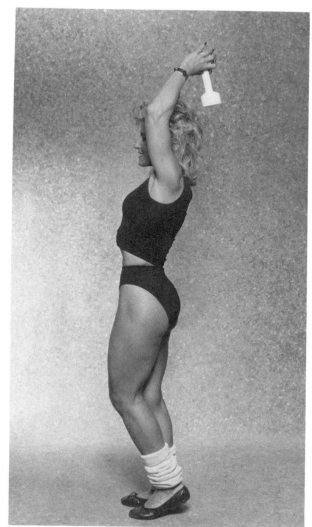

DOUBLE-ARM ID OVERHEAD EXTENSION
START

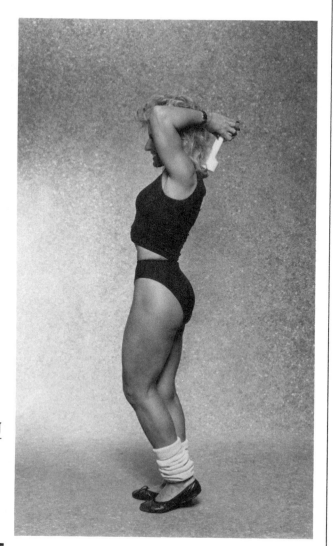

DOUBLE-ARM ID OVERHEAD EXTENSION
FINISH

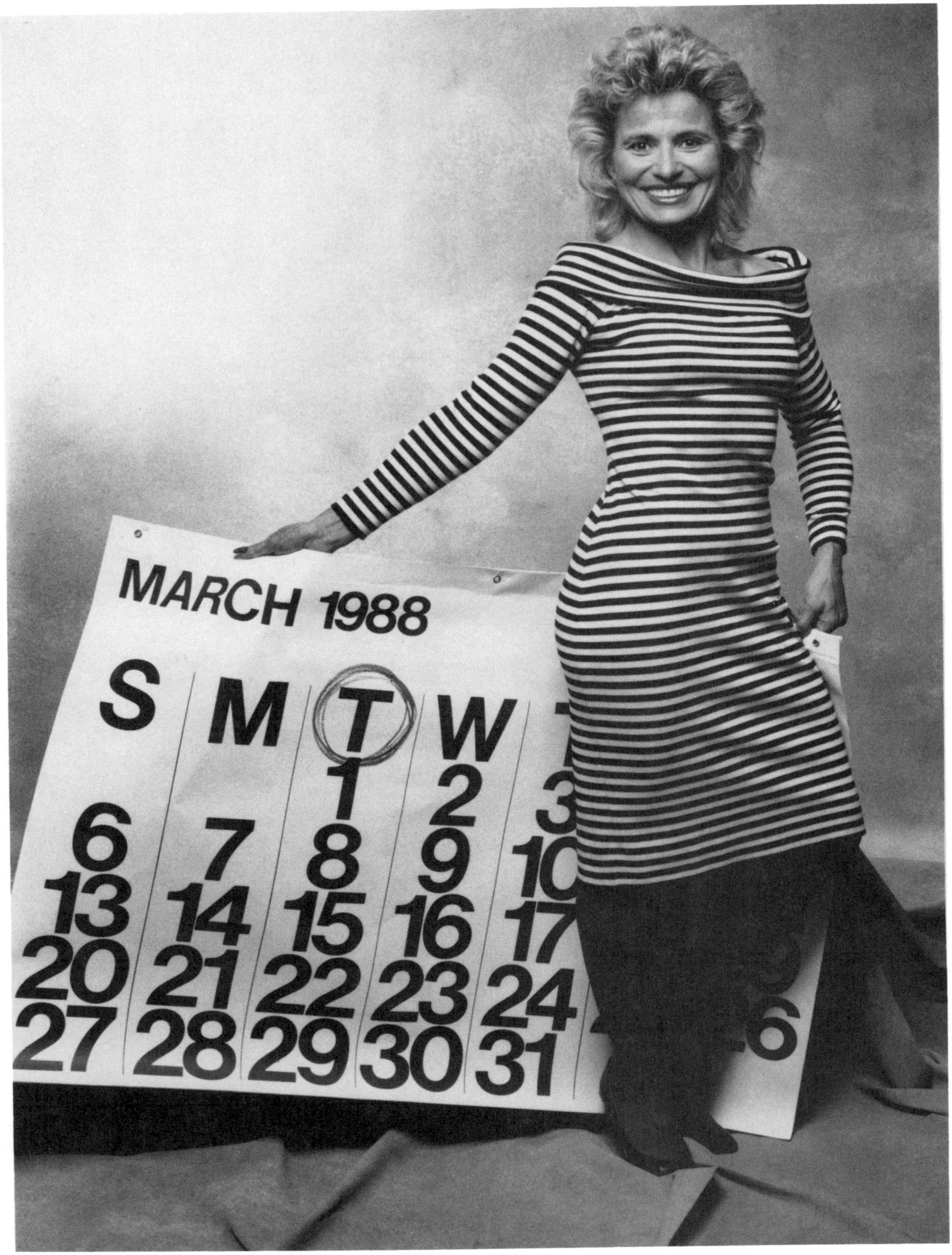
MARCH 1988
S M T W
1 2 3
6 7 8 9 10
13 14 15 16 17
20 21 22 23 24
27 28 29 30 31

5

THE 12-MINUTE TUESDAY WORKOUT

Today you're going to exercise three body parts: thighs, buttocks, and abdominals. You will do two exercises for each of them.

THIGHS: Fingertip ID squats ("squats")

Dumbbell ID lunges ("lunges")

BUTTOCKS: Dumbbell ID standing squeezes ("standing butt squeezes")

Kneeling ID angled leg lifts ("angled lifts")

ABDOMINALS: Dumbbell ID sit-ups ("sit-ups")

Dumbbell ID leg raises ("leg raises")

SETS AND REPETITIONS: Do three sets of 10 to 15 repetitions for each exercise.

EQUIPMENT: A set of three-pound dumbbells

The floor

FINGERTIP ID SQUATS– LEG EXERCISE #1

("SQUATS")

Develops: Front thigh (quadriceps) muscle and buttocks.

READY

Stand straight, with your feet shoulder-width apart and with your toes angled very slightly outward.

SET

Place your fingertips on your front thigh (quadriceps) muscle and flex (squeeze) your quadriceps so that you feel the muscle with your fingertips.

GO

Applying dynamic tension, begin descending into a squat position. As you descend, you may rise up on your toes in order to maintain your balance. Apply the full force of isometric pressure as you rise to start—all the time pressing your fingers into your tightened quadriceps muscle. Repeat the movement without letting up on the pressure and tension—until you have finished your set. Complete your final two sets and immediately move to the next exercise.

ATTENTION

Do not attempt more than 10 repetitions until you have been working out a month. By then you will have gotten used to the program and will be able to do the extra five reps without it costing too much time.

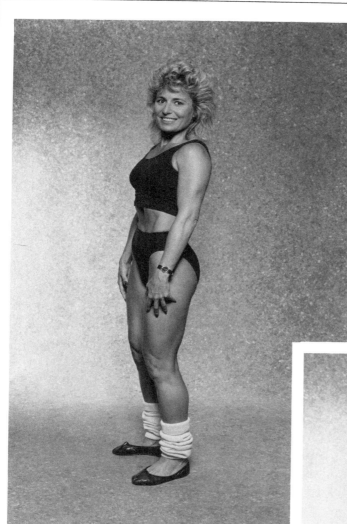

FINGERTIP ID SQUAT
START

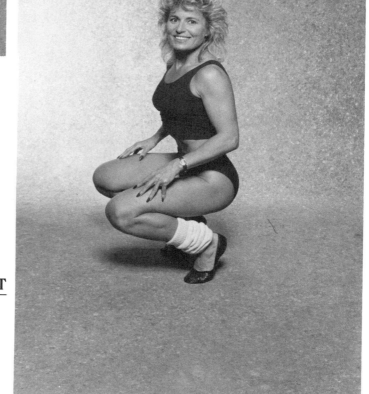

FINGERTIP ID SQUAT
FINISH

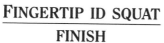

DUMBBELL ID LUNGES— LEG EXERCISE #2

("LUNGES")

Develops: Front thigh (quadriceps), hips, and buttocks.

READY

Stand straight with a three-pound dumbbell in each hand.

SET

Place your feet a natural width apart and look straight ahead.

GO

Applying dynamic tension, lunge forward with your right leg about two to three feet, letting your left knee bend so that it grazes the floor. In this position, apply the full force of dynamic tension to your stretched left leg. As you rise to start position, apply isometric pressure, and flex your quadriceps muscle when you reach start position. Repeat the movement for the other leg and continue lunging until you have finished your set. Complete your final two sets and immediately move to the next exercise.

ATTENTION

Much of the work of this exercise takes place as you rise from the down position. In order to get the maximum squeeze in the working leg, you will have to press your toes into the ground. This will provide additional pressure on the working muscle.

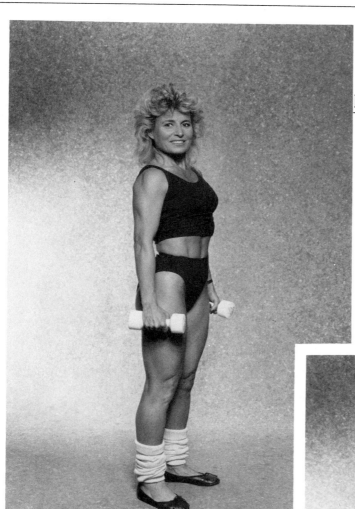

DUMBBELL ID LUNGE
START

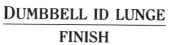

DUMBBELL ID LUNGE
FINISH

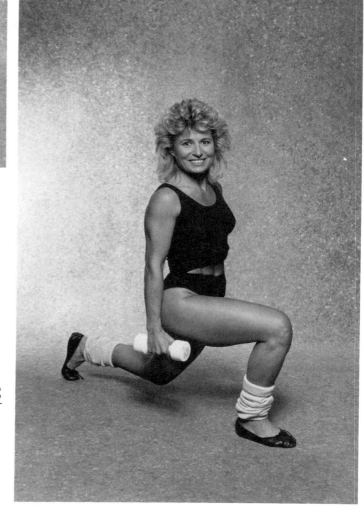

DUMBBELL STANDING ID SQUEEZES– BUTTOCKS EXERCISE #1
("STANDING BUTT SQUEEZES")

Develops: Entire buttocks area.

READY

Stand with your feet shoulder-width apart, holding a three-pound dumbbell in each hand, palms facing your body.

SET

Lower your body about four inches by bending at the knee.

GO

Squeezing your entire buttocks area as hard as possible, rise until your knees are practically locked, but, as you rise, thrust your hips slightly forward. When you reach the up position, squeeze your buttocks as hard as possible, then, applying dynamic tension, lower yourself to start position. Repeat the movement until you have finished your set. Complete your final two sets and immediately move to the next exercise.

ATTENTION

It is crucial that you continually apply isometric pressure on the up movement and dynamic tension on the down movement. The buttocks muscles should remain active throughout the exercise.

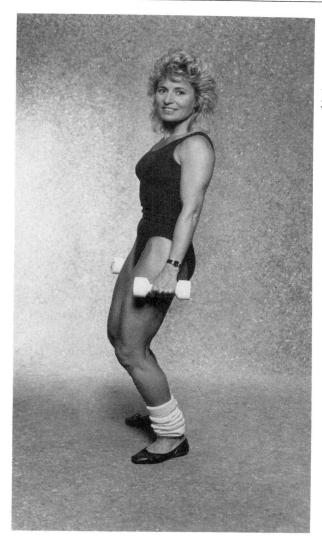

DUMBBELL STANDING ID SQUEEZE
START

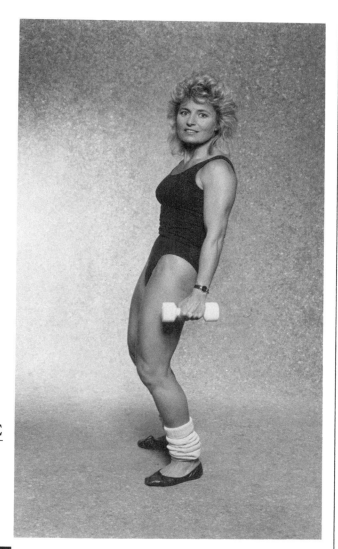

DUMBBELL STANDING ID SQUEEZE
FINISH

KNEELING ID ANGLED LEG LIFTS— BUTTOCKS EXERCISE #2
("ANGLED LIFTS")

Develops: Entire buttocks area.

READY

Take an "all-fours" position on the floor.

SET

Extend your left leg straight out behind you; point your toes back as far as possible and slightly angle them toward your body.

GO

Squeezing your left buttock as hard as possible, and keeping your left knee locked, raise your left leg as high as possible but, instead of going straight up, move your leg slightly toward your body. When your leg reaches its high position, the toes of your left foot should be in line with your kneeling right leg (see photograph). Applying the full force of dynamic tension, return to start and repeat the movement until you have finished your set. Perform the exercise for the other leg and complete your final two sets.

ATTENTION

This exercise works wonders on the buttocks area *if* you squeeze your buttocks on the upward movement as you apply isometric pressure and maintain the work on the downward movement as you apply dynamic tension. In order to see how effective the exercise is, place your left hand on your left buttock as you lift and squeeze. You'll be amazed to find that every angle of the buttock—upper, outer, inner, and lower—is being challenged simultaneously.

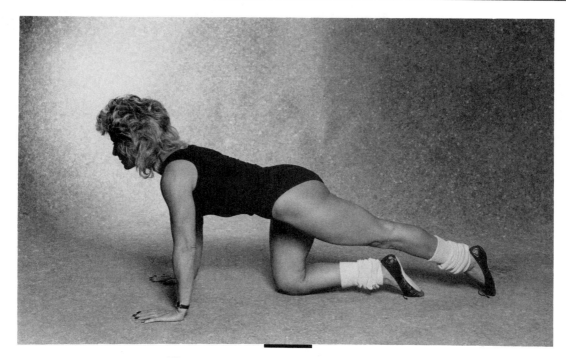

KNEELING ID ANGLED LEG-LIFT
START

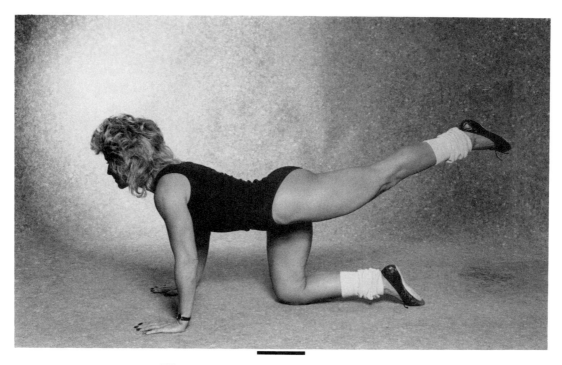

KNEELING ID ANGLED LEG-LIFT
FINISH

DUMBBELL ID SIT-UPS– ABDOMINAL EXERCISE #1
("SIT-UPS")

Develops: Upper abdominal area.

READY

Lie on the floor with one dumbbell placed on your upper abdominal area.

SET

Place one hand on the dumbbell and one hand behind your head, and bend your knees very slightly. If there is an available chair or couch, you can place your feet under it—but it is not necessary. You can cross your legs at the ankles instead.

GO

Squeezing your upper abdominal area as hard as possible, and applying isometric pressure, rise to a sitting position. Apply dynamic tension as you return to start and repeat the movement until you have completed your set. Switch the arm that is holding the dumbbell and do your next set. For your final set, do five repetitions with one arm holding the dumbbell and five with the other arm holding the dumbbell.

ATTENTION

The arm-switching is necessary in order to ensure even development of your abdominal muscles.

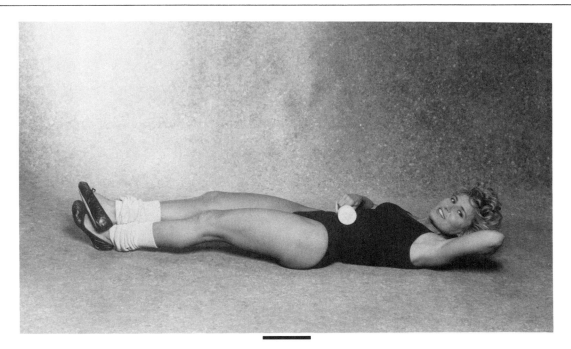

DUMBBELL ID SIT-UP
START

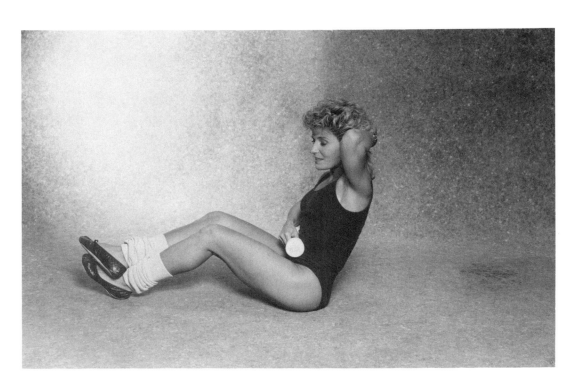

DUMBBELL ID SIT-UP
FINISH

DUMBBELL ID LEG RAISES–
ABDOMINAL EXERCISE #2
("LEG RAISES")

Develops: Lower abdominal area.

READY

Lie on the floor and place a three-pound dumbbell between your feet.

SET

Place your shoulders firmly on the ground and bend your knees very slightly. Place your hands behind your neck.

GO

Squeeze your lower abdominal area as hard as possible and, applying isometric pressure, raise your legs until they are perpendicular to the floor. Apply dynamic tension as you return to start position. With no rest and no lessening of the tension and pressure, repeat the movement until you have finished your set. Complete your final two sets.

ATTENTION

Don't get so carried away with squeezing your abdominal muscles that you forget to secure the three-pound dumbbell between your feet. Even though it's light, it can do damage if it falls on your nose.

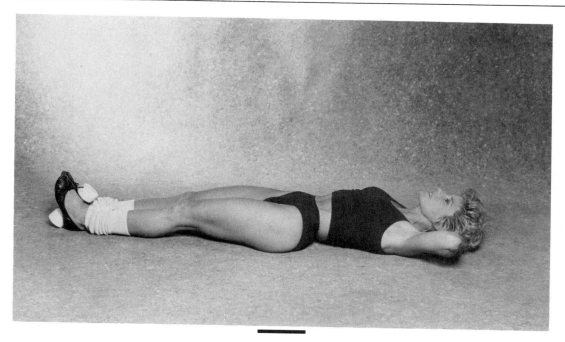

DUMBBELL ID LEG-RAISE
START

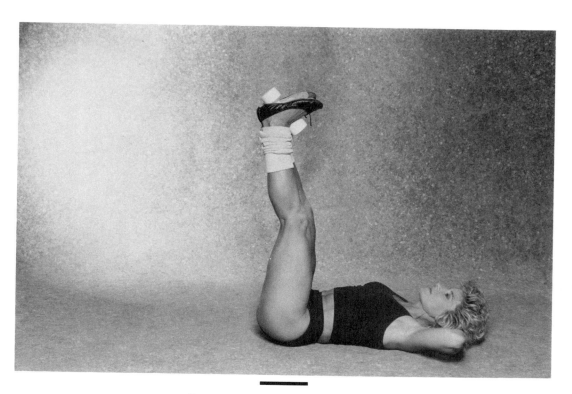

DUMBBELL ID LEG-RAISE
FINISH

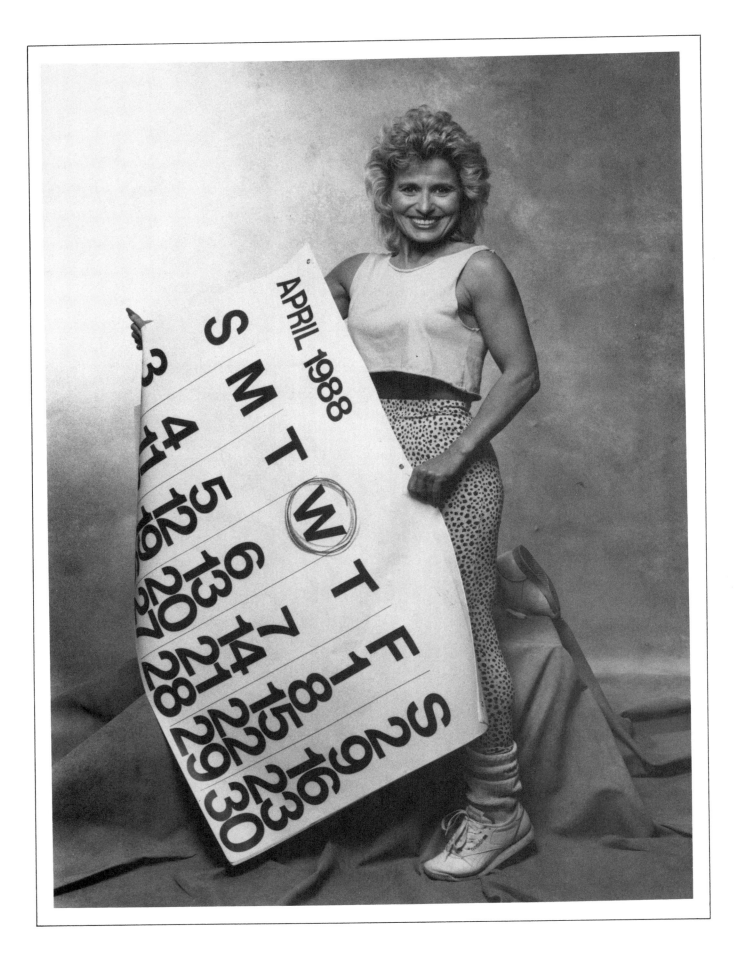

6

THE 12-MINUTE WEDNESDAY WOROUT

Today you're going to exercise three body parts: back, biceps, and calves. You will do two exercises for back and biceps, and one exercise for calves.

BACK: Seated ID back laterals ("back laterals")

Standing ID leaning pulls ("leaning pulls")

BICEPS: Seated alternate ID dumbbell curls ("alternate curls")

Leaning ID concentration curls ("concentrations")

CALVES: Seated ID calf raises ("seated raises")

SETS AND
REPETITIONS: Do three sets of 10 repetitions for each exercise.

EQUIPMENT: A set of three-pound dumbbells

A chair

A telephone directory, thick book, or attaché case

SEATED ID BACK LATERALS– BACK EXERCISE #1
("BACK LATERALS")

Develops: Upper back and trapezius muscles.

READY

Sit at the edge of a chair, holding a three-pound dumbbell in each hand, palms facing behind you.

SET

Lean over until your chest touches your knees. Let the dumbbells pull your arms into a fully extended, relaxed position.

GO

Applying isometric pressure, squeeze your upper back muscles and raise your arms up and back while rotating the dumbbells so that your palms face forward. Continue to raise the dumbbells until they reach hip level, keeping your elbows close to your sides at all times. Squeeze your shoulders together when you reach the up position. Apply dynamic tension as you return to start position and repeat the movement until you have finished your set. Complete your final two sets, shrug your shoulders a few times, and immediately move to the next exercise.

ATTENTION

You can prevent your back muscles from feeling cramped by stretching your arms as low to the floor as possible on the down movement.

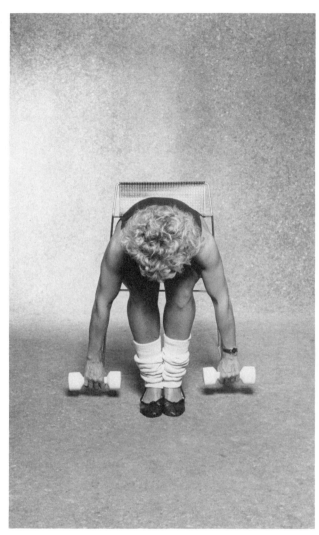

SEATED ID BACK LATERAL
START

SEATED ID BACK LATERAL
FINISH

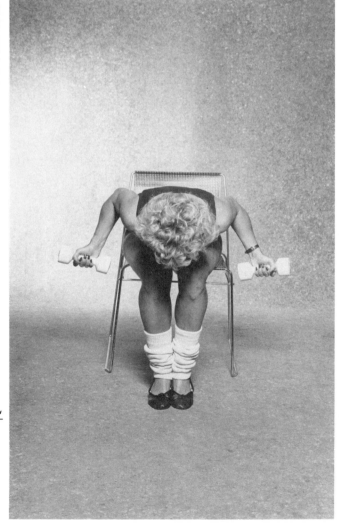

STANDING ID LEANING PULLS—BACK EXERCISE #2

("LEANING PULLS")

Develops: Latissimus dorsi muscles—"lats"—and upper back muscles.

READY

Stand with a three-pound dumbbell in each hand, palms facing behind you.

SET

Lean over slightly and raise your arms straight up so that your biceps are in line with, and about four inches away from, your mouth-nose area.

GO

Applying isometric pressure, squeeze your upper back and lat muscles and, keeping your elbows locked, begin lowering your arms until the dumbbells reach your back thigh area. Apply dynamic tension as you return to start position. Repeat the movement until you have finished your set. Complete your final two sets, shake out your back and immediately move to the next exercise.

ATTENTION

Do not arch your back as you lean forward. Keep it straight. This exercise is very effective if you maintain the correct position. (See photograph.)

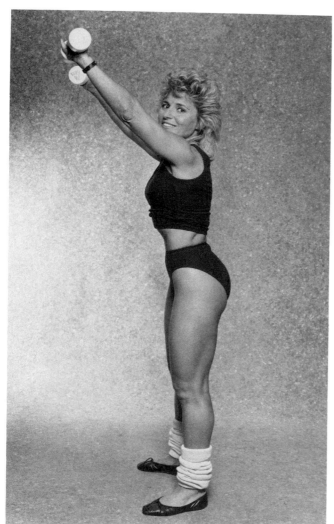

STANDING ID LEANING PULL
START

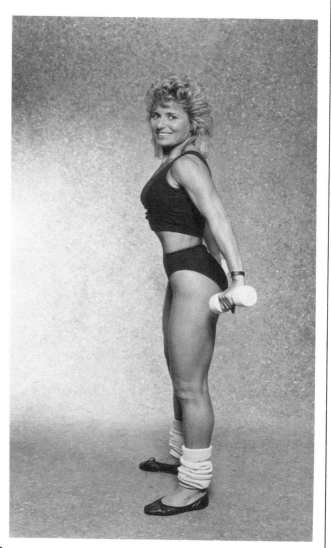

STANDING ID LEANING PULL
FINISH

SEATED ALTERNATE ID DUMBBELL CURLS—BICEPS EXERCISE #1

("ALTERNATE CURLS")

Develops: Biceps and forearm.

READY

Sit at the edge of a chair holding a three-pound dumbbell in each hand, palms facing away from your body.

SET

Let your arms hang straight down, and keep your elbows close to your body. Curl your wrists slightly inward and lock them.

GO

Apply isometric pressure as you flex your biceps as hard as possible and begin raising your right arm to shoulder height. As you lower your right arm to start position, apply dynamic tension, and at the same time start curling your left arm to the up position. Continue to raise and lower the dumbbells alternately until you have completed 10 repetitions for each arm. Complete your final two sets, shake out your arms, and immediately move to the next exercise.

ATTENTION

Beware of the temptation to let up on the isometric pressure and dynamic tension during this exercise. Watch your biceps muscles as they contract and expand with each movement.

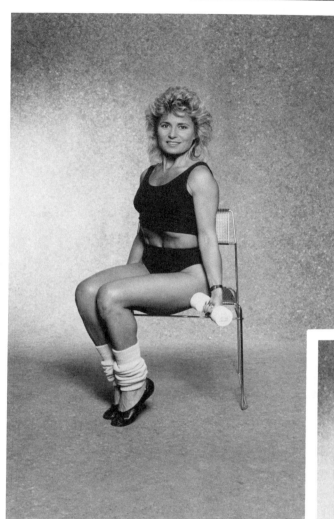

SEATED ALTERNATE ID DUMBBELL CURL
START

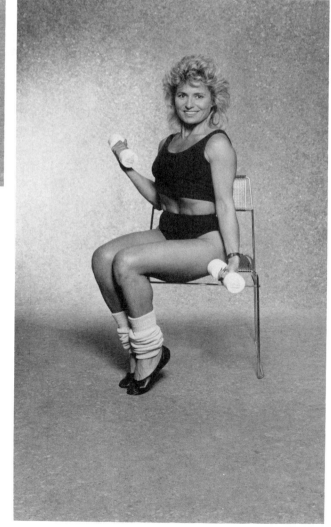

SEATED ALTERNATE ID DUMBBELL CURL
FINISH

LEANING ID CONCENTRATION CURLS–BICEPS EXERCISE #2

("CONCENTRATIONS")

Develops: The entire biceps muscle.

READY

Stand with one three-pound dumbbell in your right hand, palm facing away from you.

SET

Lean over until your left knee is about three inches off the ground. Place your right elbow on your right inner knee, letting the dumbbell hang straight down, and place your left hand on your left thigh for support. The position may seem awkward at first, but you'll quickly adjust to it.

GO

Apply isometric pressure to your right biceps as you curl your arm up until you cannot go any higher. Keep your wrist locked and slightly curled toward your body. Apply dynamic tension as you return to start position. Repeat the movement until you have completed 10 repetitions. Switch to your left arm and do 10 repetitions. Continue alternating arms until you have finished all three sets. Shake out your arms and immediately move to the next exercise.

ATTENTION

Keep your eye on your working biceps. You will clearly see how the muscle is being challenged. Concentrate all of your mental and physical energy on that working muscle.

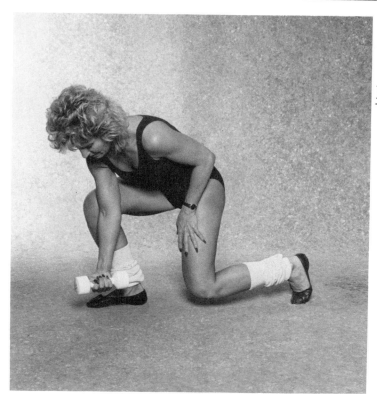

LEANING ID CONCENTRATION CURL
START

LEANING ID CONCENTRATION CURL
FINISH

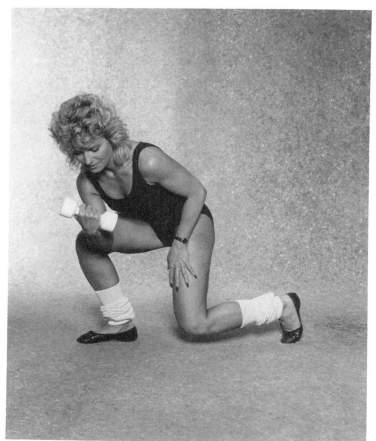

SEATED ID CALF RAISES– CALF EXERCISE #1
("SEATED RAISES")

Develops: Calf (gastrocnemius) muscle.

READY

Sit at the edge of a chair with your back straight and your feet on top of a telephone directory, thick book, or attaché case.

SET

Place a three-pound dumbbell between your knees and hold it there with pressure. Place the balls of your feet on the telephone directory, with your toes pointed straight ahead. Lower your heels an inch or two toward the ground.

GO

Applying isometric pressure, raise your heels until your feet are resting on the balls of the feet. Go as high as possible. Apply dynamic tension as you return to start position. Repeat the movement until you have finished your set. Complete your final two sets and shake out your calves.

ATTENTION

You may get a momentary cramp in your calves if you are not used to working these muscles. If this happens, stop exercising and bounce on the ball of your foot a few times. Then continue the exercise, but do not apply quite as much pressure. You may have to apply moderate pressure at first and gradually increase it as you get used to the exercise.

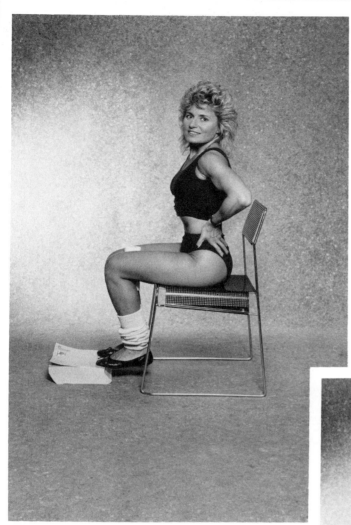

SEATED ID CALF RAISE
START

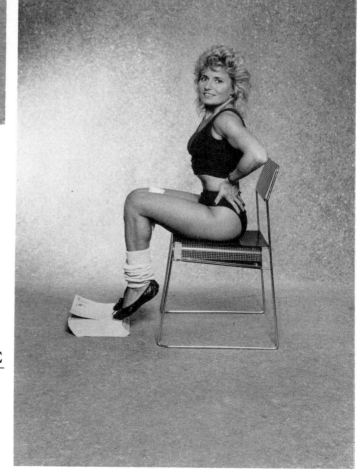

SEATED ID CALF RAISE
FINISH

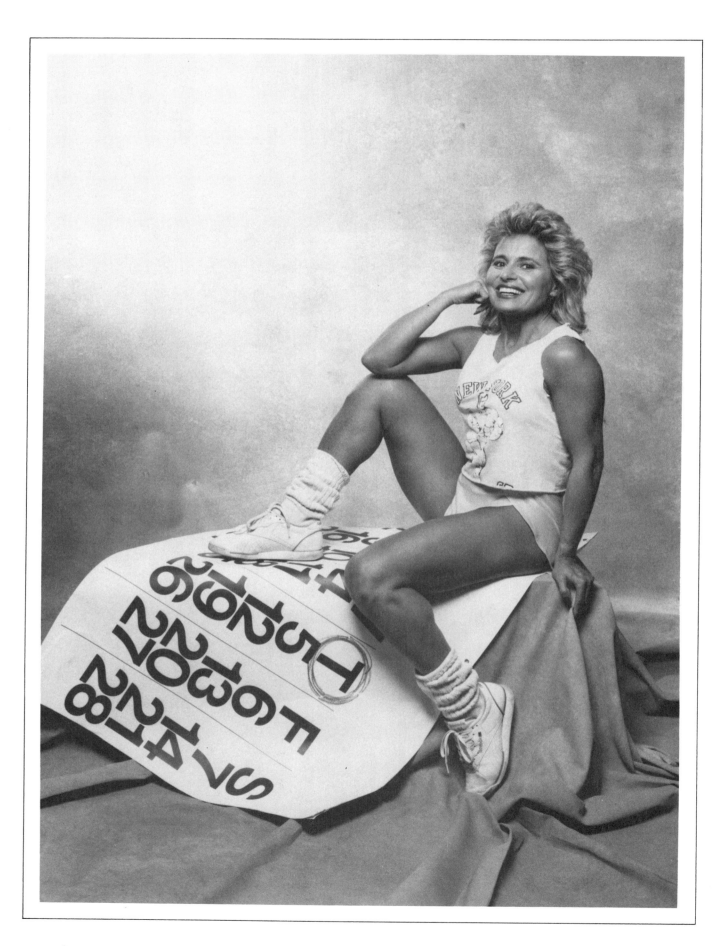

7

THE 12-MINUTE
THURSDAY WORKOUT

Today you're going to exercise three body parts: chest, shoulders, and triceps. You will do three exercises for each of them. This is your second weekly workout for those body parts (you already worked on them on Monday). The exercises you will do today are not the same as the ones you did on Monday, because, in order to ensure perfectly balanced muscular development, it's necessary to perform a variety of exercises for the same muscle, and to exercise the muscles from various angles.

CHEST: Standing ID dumbbell crossovers ("crossovers")

Seated ID dumbbell chest squeezes ("pec squeezes")

SHOULDERS: Standing ID side lateral raises ("side laterals")

Bent-over ID lateral raises ("bent laterals")

TRICEPS: Kneeling ID dumbbell pulldowns
("kneeling triceps pulldowns")

Standing ID dumbbell pushdowns ("pushdowns")

SETS AND
REPETITIONS: Do three sets of 10 repetitions for each exercise.

EQUIPMENT: A set of three-pound dumbbells

A chair

STANDING ID DUMBBELL CROSSOVERS—CHEST EXERCISE #1

("CROSSOVERS")

Develops: Inner and lower area of pectoral muscle.

READY

Stand in a natural position, holding a three-pound dumbbell in each hand, palms facing your sides.

SET

Extend your arms outward at your sides until they are higher than ear height. Curve your wrists slightly downward and lock them.

GO

Apply isometric pressure to your chest (pectoral) muscles and, keeping your arms in a slightly bent position, lower the dumbbells until they nearly touch at the center of your body. Crunch your pectoral muscles together. Applying dynamic tension and stretching your pectoral muscles, return to start position. Repeat the movement until you have finished your set. Complete your final two sets, shrug your shoulders a few times, and immediately move to the next exercise.

ATTENTION

Don't rock back and forth as you lower and raise the dumbbells. Your head, torso, and legs should remain absolutely still—the only part of your body moving should be your arms. Keep your mind on your chest (pectoral) muscles throughout the movement.

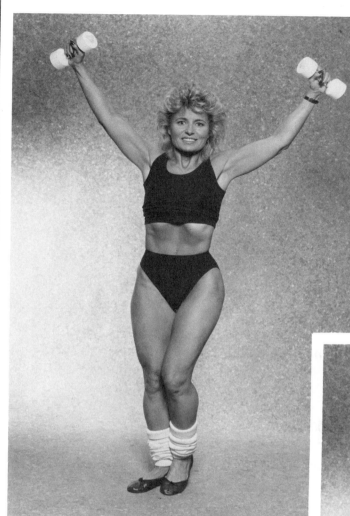

STANDING ID DUMBBELL CROSSOVER
START

STANDING ID DUMBBELL CROSSOVER
FINISH

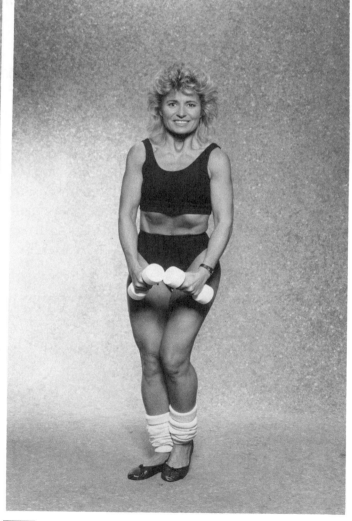

SEATED ID DUMBBELL CHEST SQUEEZES—CHEST EXERCISE #2
("PEC SQUEEZES")

Develops: Entire pectoral muscle, especially the inner area.

READY

Sit on a chair, holding a three-pound dumbbell in each hand.

SET

Raise your arms to form two "Ls" by bending your elbows and extending your arms outward. The dumbbells are held palms outward, in a horizontal position.

GO

Apply isometric pressure as you move your arms toward your chest, all the time maintaining the "L" position of your arms. Continue to move your elbows toward your chest until your forearms are about eight inches apart and your elbows are in line with your breasts. Apply dynamic tension as you return to start position, stretching your pectoral muscles as you reach start. Without resting, repeat the movement until you have finished your set. Complete your final two sets, shrug your shoulders a few times, and immediately move to the next exercise.

ATTENTION

It is crucial that you maintain the "L" position of your arms throughout the exercise.

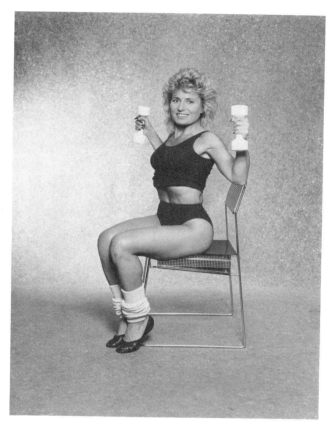

SEATED ID DUMBBELL CHEST SQUEEZE
START

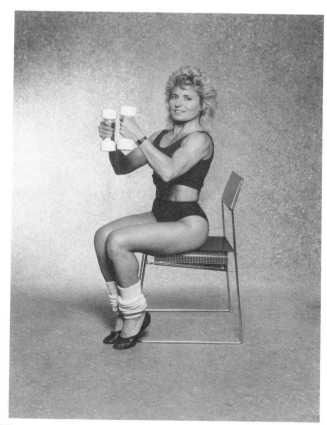

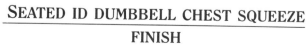

SEATED ID DUMBBELL CHEST SQUEEZE
FINISH

STANDING ID SIDE LATERAL RAISES– SHOULDER EXERCISE #1
("SIDE LATERALS")

Develops: The side (medial) shoulder (deltoid) muscle.

READY

Stand in a natural position with a three-pound dumbbell in each hand, palms facing each other.

SET

Let the dumbbells touch your thighs and lean very slightly forward.

GO

Squeeze your side (medial) shoulder area and raise the dumbbells outward, leading with your locked outer wrists and elbows, until the dumbbells reach ear height. Your elbows will be slightly bent in this position. Apply dynamic tension as you return to start position, and repeat the movement until you have finished your set. Complete your final two sets, shake out your shoulder-to-wrist area, and immediately move to the next exercise.

ATTENTION

Do not rock back and forth as you move the dumbbells. The only body parts moving are your arms. Focus your mind strictly on the medial deltoids as you exercise.

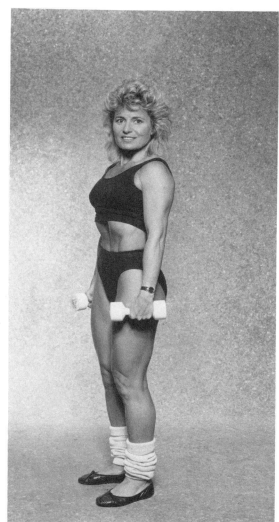

STANDING ID SIDE LATERAL RAISE
START

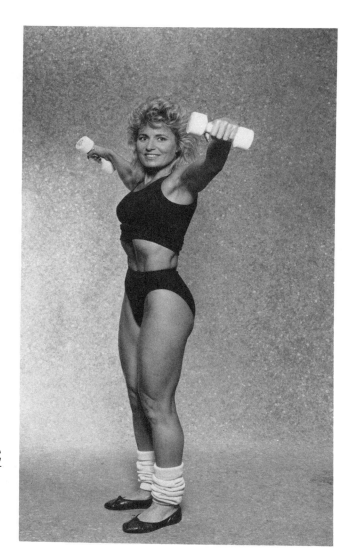

STANDING ID SIDE LATERAL RAISE
FINISH

BENT-OVER ID LATERAL RAISES– SHOULDER EXERCISE #2
("BENT LATERALS")

Develops: Rear (posterior) and side (medial)
shoulder (deltoid) muscles.

READY

Stand in a natural position with a three-pound dumbbell in each hand, palms facing inward.

SET

Lean over until your torso is parallel to the floor; let the dumbbells touch each other at the center of your body.

GO

Flex your shoulder muscles and, squeezing as hard as possible, extend your arms outward until they are nearly parallel to the floor. Your elbows should be very slightly bent in this position. Apply the full force of dynamic tension as you return to start position and repeat the movement until you have finished your set. Complete your final two sets, shrug your shoulders a few times, and immediately move to the next exercise.

ATTENTION

Beware of the temptation to rise from the bent-over position as you are working. Maintain your torso parallel to the floor throughout the movement. Keep your mind on your rear deltoid muscles throughout the movement.

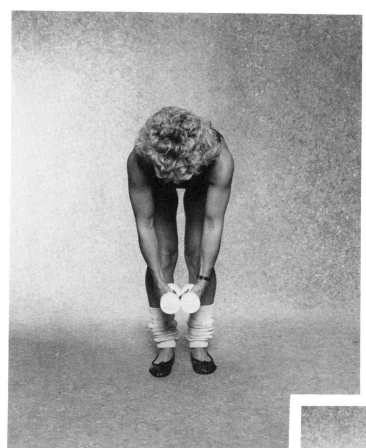

BENT-OVER ID LATERAL RAISE
START

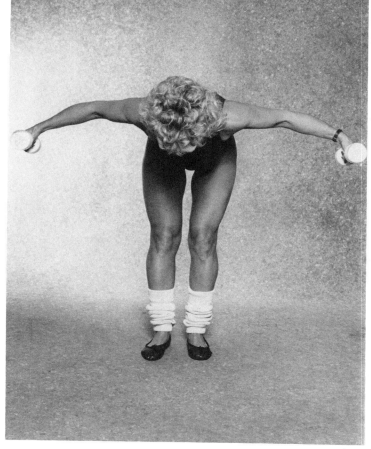

BENT-OVER ID LATERAL RAISE
FINISH

KNEELING ID DUMBBELL PULLDOWNS—TRICEPS EXERCISE #1
("KNEELING TRICEPS PULLDOWNS")

Develops: The entire triceps area, especially the
inner head of the muscle.

READY

Kneel on the floor, holding a three-pound dumbbell in each hand, palms
facing each other.

SET

Bend your elbows and let the dumbbells touch at the center of your chest
area. Lean slightly forward. You are in a "praying" position.

GO

Keeping your upper arms as close to your body as possible and using
isometric pressure, lower the dumbbells until your arms are extended
straight down, and then turn your wrists outward and squeeze as hard as
possible. Apply dynamic tension as you return to the start position, and
repeat the movement until you have finished your set. Complete your final
two sets, shake out your arms, and immediately move to the next exercise.

ATTENTION

Keep your mind on your triceps muscles while performing this exercise. As
you reach the down-back position, flex your triceps muscle for a split second
before applying dynamic tension as you return to start.

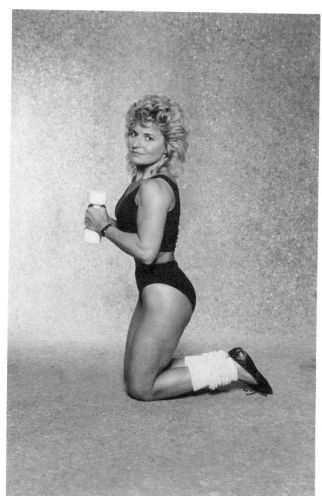

KNEELING ID DUMBBELL PULLDOWN
START

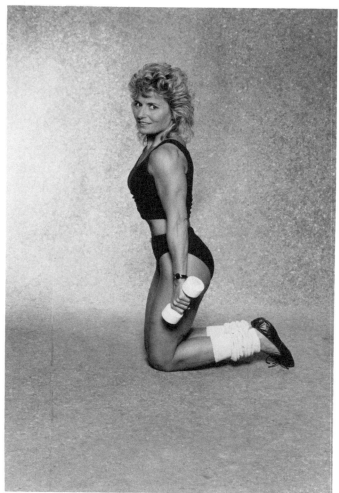

KNEELING ID DUMBBELL PULLDOWN
FINISH

STANDING ID DUMBBELL PUSHDOWNS—TRICEPS EXERCISE #2
("PUSHDOWNS")

Develops: The entire triceps area, especially the
outer head of the muscle.

READY

Stand in a natural position with one dumbbell held with both hands.

SET

Bend your elbows and pin them to your side. The dumbbell should be held
palms down and should be held just about chest height. Lock your wrists.

GO

Keeping your upper arms as close to your body as possible, begin applying
isometric pressure as you lower your arms until they are fully extended
downward. The dumbbell should nearly touch your front thigh area on the
down position. Apply dynamic tension as you raise the dumbbell to start
position. Repeat the movement until you have finished your set. Complete
your final two sets and shake out your arms.

ATTENTION

Be sure to keep your elbows close to your sides throughout the movement.
Imagine them riveted to your waist area.

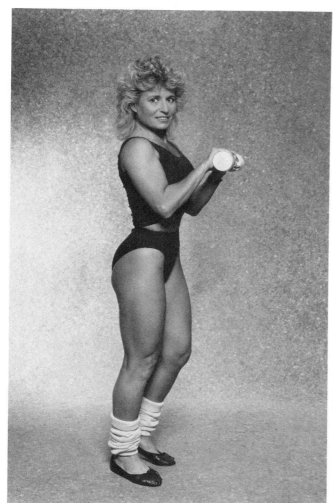

STANDING ID DUMBBELL PUSHDOWN
START

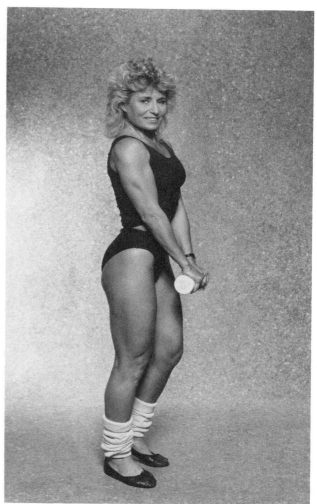

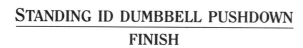

STANDING ID DUMBBELL PUSHDOWN
FINISH

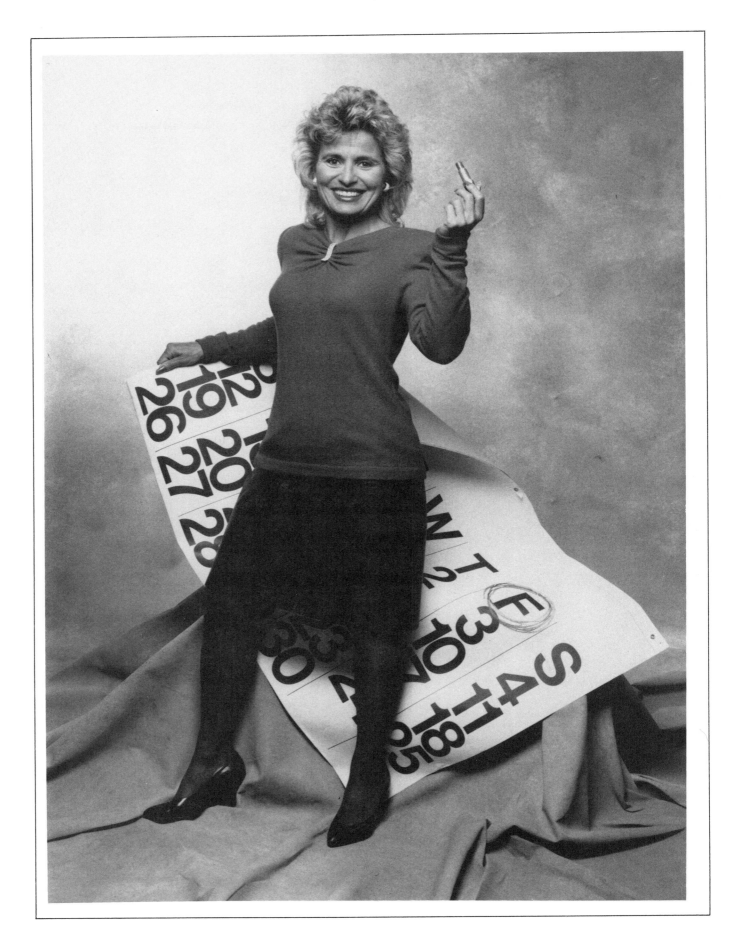

8

THE 12-MINUTE FRIDAY WORKOUT

Today you will perform your second weekly exercises for your thighs, buttocks, and abdominals—but because muscles need a variety of exercises in order to develop into perfect form, you will not do the same exercises for these body parts that you did on Tuesday.

THIGHS: Seated ID leg extensions ("extensions")

Lying ID leg curls ("leg curls")

BUTTOCKS: Seated ID scissors ("scissors")

Kneeling ID feather kick-ups ("feathers")

ABDOMINALS: Seated ID leg-ins ("leg-ins")

ID crunch twists ("crunch twists")

SETS AND REPETITIONS: Do three sets of 10 to 15 repetitions.

EQUIPMENT: A set of three-pound dumbbells

A chair

SEATED ID LEG EXTENSIONS– THIGH EXERCISE #1
("EXTENSIONS")

Develops: Front thigh (quadriceps) muscle.

READY

Sit at the edge of a chair with your feet on the ground and a three-pound dumbbell held between your feet.

SET

Hold on to the chair on either side of you; lean back about six inches and arch your back slightly.

GO

Tense your quadriceps muscles and extend your legs straight out in front of you until your knees are locked. Apply dynamic tension as you return to start position. Repeat the movement until you have finished your set. Complete your final two sets, shake out each leg, and immediately move to the next exercise.

ATTENTION

Be sure to apply the maximum amount of isometric pressure as you extend your legs, and the full amount of dynamic tension as you return to start position. Keep your mind on your quadriceps muscle throughout the movement.

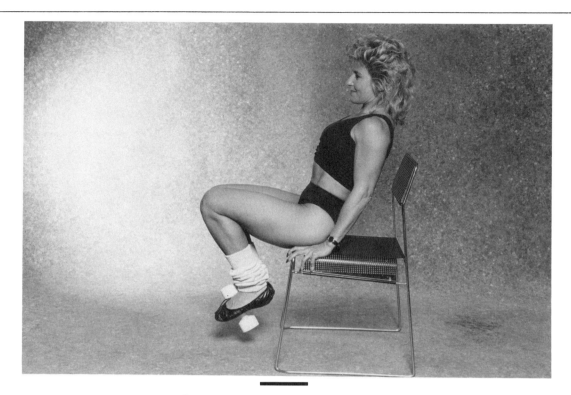

SEATED ID LEG EXTENSION
START

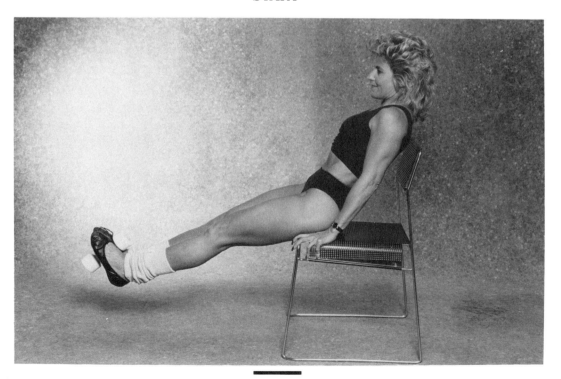

SEATED ID LEG EXTENSION
FINISH

LYING ID LEG CURLS— THIGH EXERCISE #2
("LEG CURLS")

Develops: Back thigh (biceps femoris) muscles,
otherwise known as the hamstrings.

READY

Lie on the floor, face down, with a dumbbell held between your feet.

SET

Place your chest flat on the ground, and place your folded hands under your chin. Secure the weight firmly between your feet.

GO

Squeeze your back thigh muscles as hard as possible and, applying isometric pressure, bend your knees and raise your lower legs until they are perpendicular to the floor. Apply dynamic tension as you return to start position. Repeat the movement until you have finished your set. Complete your final two sets, shake out each leg, and immediately move to the next exercise.

ATTENTION

In order to get the maximum isometric pressure and dynamic tension, press your heel-to-ankle area tightly together as you raise and lower your legs. This will also help to keep the weight in place.

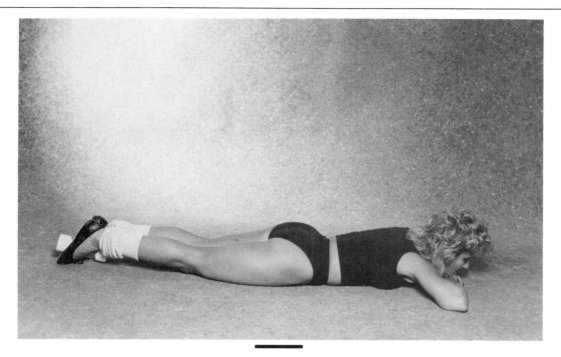

LYING ID LEG CURL
START

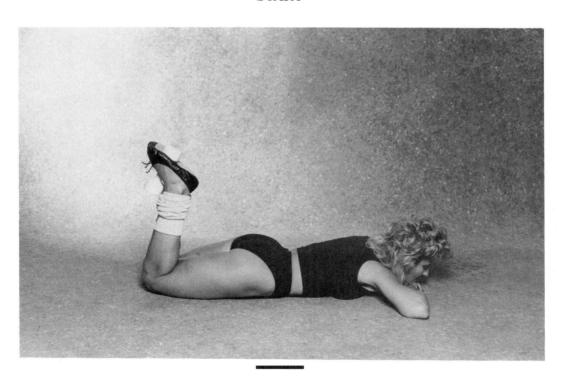

LYING ID LEG CURL
FINISH

Seated ID Scissors– Buttocks Exercise #1

("SCISSORS")

Develops: Entire buttocks area.

READY

Sit at the edge of a chair and place one hand under each buttock.

SET

Lean back until your back touches the chair back and extend your legs straight out in front of your. Lock your knees.

GO

Squeeze your entire buttocks area as hard as possible. (You can feel your buttocks tighten with your hands.) Apply isometric pressure as you scissor your legs apart as wide as they can go. Apply dynamic tension as you return to start position, and repeat the movement until you have finished your set. Complete your final two sets. Stand up and shake your buttocks a few times, then immediately move to the next exercise.

ATTENTION

It is crucial that you remember to apply the pressure to your buttocks and not to your thighs when performing this exercise. Remember: Pay attention to the body part you are working—and to that body part alone.

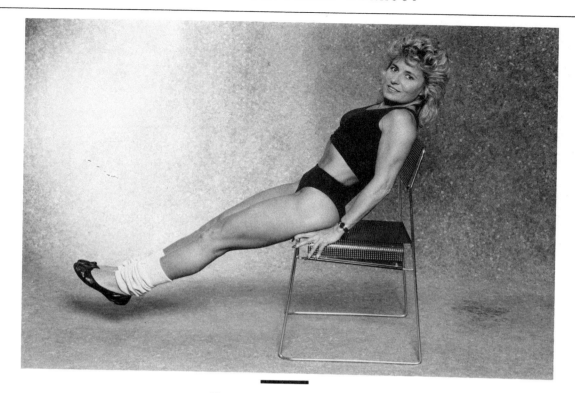

SEATED ID SCISSOR
START

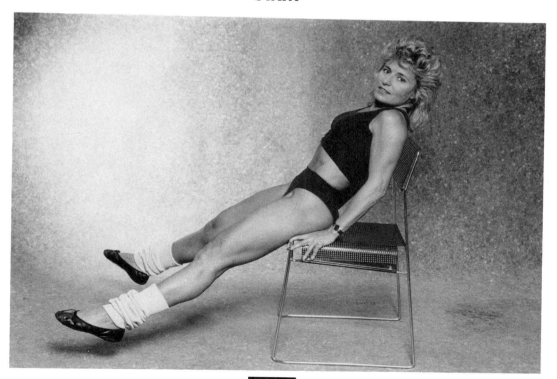

SEATED ID SCISSOR
FINISH

KNEELING ID FEATHER KICK-UPS– BUTTOCKS EXERCISE #2

("FEATHERS")

Develops: Entire buttocks area.

READY

Take an "all-fours" position on the floor.

SET

Raise your left thigh up and bend your knee so that your leg takes the shape of an "L."

GO

Squeeze your buttocks as hard as possible and apply isometric pressure as you extend your right buttock-to-thigh area as high as possible, until your leg is extended straight upward and as high as possible. Point your toe. Apply dynamic tension as you return to start position, and repeat the movement until you have completed your set. Switch to the other leg and perform your set. Continue to move from right to left leg until you have completed all three sets. Jump up and down on each leg a few times, letting your buttocks bounce, and immediately move to the next exercise.

ATTENTION

Be careful to maintain the "L" bend whenever you return to start position. You will have to do the exercise very slowly in the beginning. If you're having trouble, isolate each repetition, making a conscious effort to return to the "L" position after each extension. This exercise is awkward at first, but after a few weeks most people find it easy to do—and they do it in perfect form. It is probably the most effective of all the buttocks exercises, so it's worth the breaking-in period.

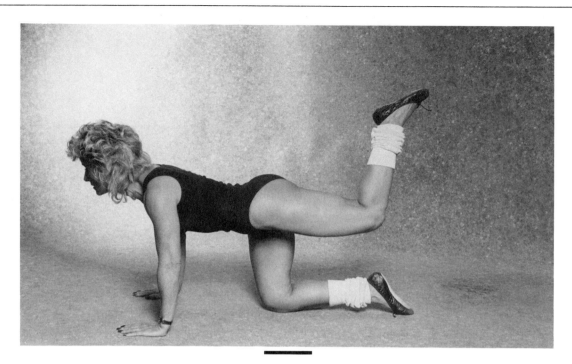

KNEELING ID FEATHER KICK-UP
START

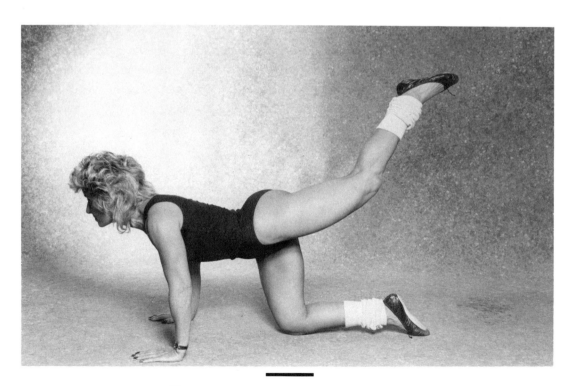

KNEELING ID FEATHER KICK-UP
FINISH

SEATED ID LEG-INS–ABDOMINAL EXERCISE #1
("LEG-INS")

Develops: Lower abdominal area.

READY

Sit at the edge of a chair with a dumbbell held between your feet.

SET

Lean back until your shoulders touch the back of the chair. Grip the chair on either side in front of you and extend your legs straight out in front.

GO

Squeeze your abdominal muscles and pull your knees toward your chest until they cannot go any farther. Apply dynamic tension as you return to start position and repeat the movement until you have finished your set. Complete your final two sets and stand up and twist your upper body a few times, then immediately move to the next exercise.

ATTENTION

This exercise tightens the entire abdominal area, but it is especially designed for that difficult-to-reach lower abdominal area. However, you must remember to focus your full attention directly on your lower abdominals for every single moment of the exercise if you want to see maximum results. If you find it awkward doing the exercise this way, try sitting at the side of the chair. You can hold on to the side of the chair with one hand, and the back of the chair with the other.

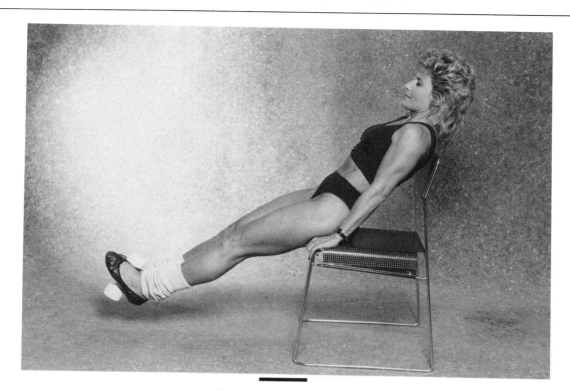

SEATED ID LEG-IN
START

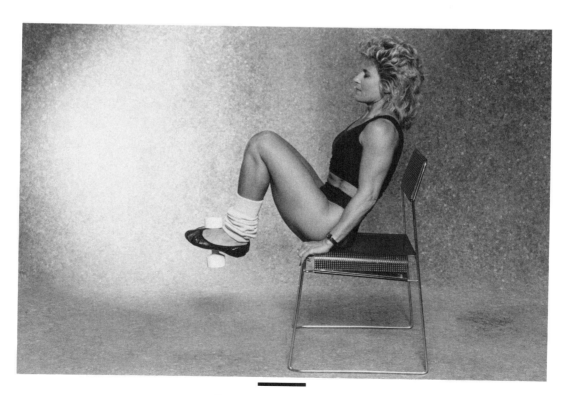

SEATED ID LEG-IN
FINISH

Id CRUNCH TWISTS–
ABDOMINAL EXERCISE #2
("CRUNCH TWISTS")

Develops: Upper abdominal area, intercostal muscles.

READY

Lie on the floor, flat on your back.

SET

Cross your legs at the ankles and bend your knees slightly. Place your hands behind your neck and interlace your fingers.

GO

Apply isometric pressure as you squeeze your abdominal muscles as hard as possible, and raise your shoulders off the floor while moving your right elbow toward your left knee. Don't allow your body to rise any higher than shoulders-off-the-floor height. Apply dynamic tension as you return to start. Then repeat the movement for the other side of your body. Continue this alternating right-left movement until you have done 10 to 15 repetitions for each side. Complete your final two sets, then stand up and jump up and down.

ATTENTION

This is not a sit-up. It's a crunch. You must not raise your body more than shoulders-off-the-floor height. Remember to keep your abdominal muscles flexed and tensed throughout the exercise. If you get a cramp, lie flat on your back and completely relax. The cramp should go away in a few seconds.

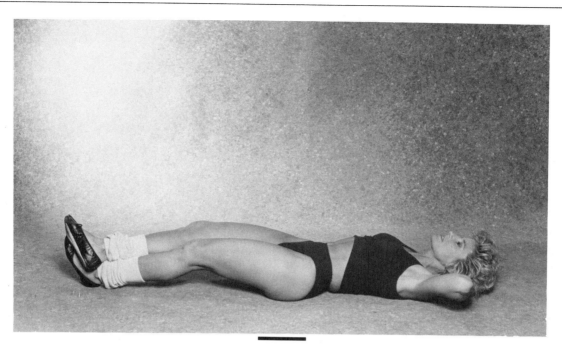

ID CRUNCH TWIST
START

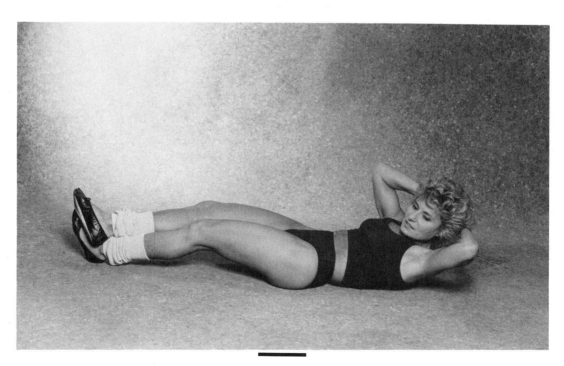

ID CRUNCH TWIST
FINISH

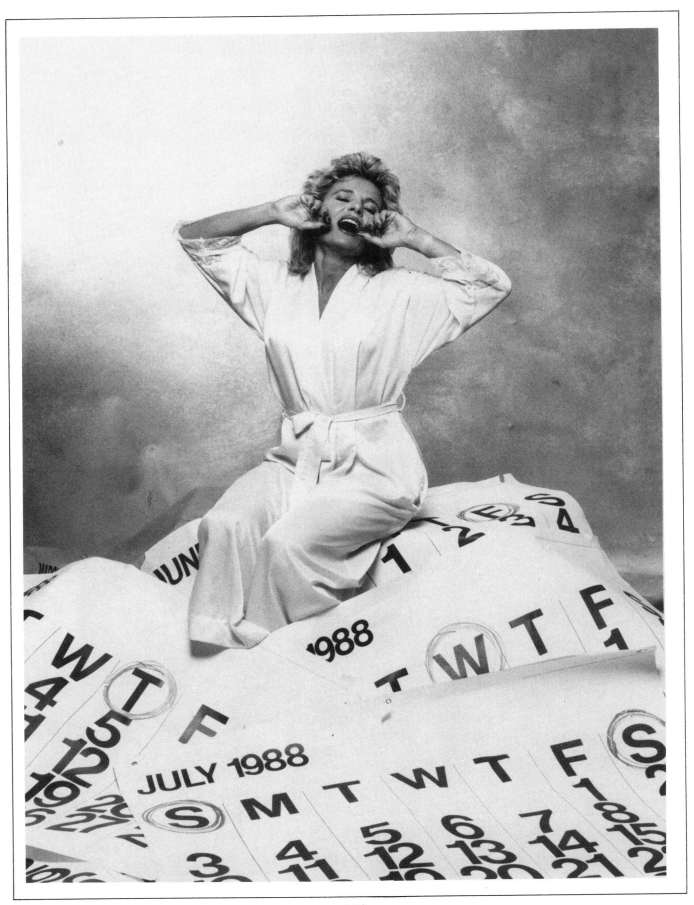

9

THE 12-MINUTE SATURDAY AND SUNDAY WORKOUT

SATURDAY

Today you will perform your second weekly exercises for your back, biceps, and calves—but you will not be doing the same exercises you did on Wednesday. Muscles need stimulation from various angles in order to develop into perfectly symmetrical form.

BACK: Bent ID dumbbell rows ("bent rows")

ID dumbbell lat pulldowns ("lat pulldowns")

BICEPS: ID dumbbell preacher curls ("preachers")

Standing simultaneous ID dumbbell curls ("simultaneous curls")

CALVES: Standing one-leg ID dumbbell calf raises ("standing raises")

SETS AND
REPETITIONS: Do three sets of 10 repetitions.

EQUIPMENT: A set of three-pound dumbbells

A chair

A telephone directory, thick book, or attaché case

BENT ID DUMBBELL ROWS–BACK EXERCISE #1

("BENT ROWS")

Develops: Latissimus dorsi ("lats") and trapezius muscles.

READY

Stand with your feet shoulder-width apart, holding a dumbbell in each hand.

SET

Hold the dumbbells palms facing inward and about six inches away from the sides of your body. Bend at the knees slightly and lean forward until your torso is slightly higher than parallel to the floor. Arch your back.

GO

Apply isometric pressure to your latissimus dorsi muscles and pull the dumbbells up until they are about waist height at the sides of your body. Apply dynamic tension and return to start position, and repeat the movement until you have finished your set. Complete your final two sets, shrug your shoulders a few times, and immediately move to the next exercise.

ATTENTION

It is crucial that you keep your mind on your latissimus dorsi muscles throughout the exercise. You should be able actually to feel your lats expanding and working on the up movement and contracting and condensing on the down movement. Remember: The power is in your concentration as you throw your mind into working your lats.

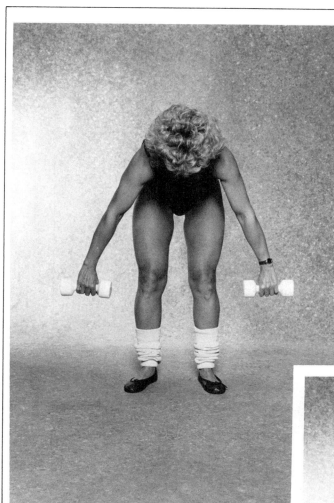

BENT ID DUMBBELL ROW
START

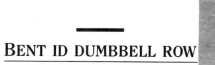

BENT ID DUMBBELL ROW
FINISH

Id DUMBBELL LAT PULLDOWNS– BACK EXERCISE #2

("LAT PULLDOWNS")

Develops: Latissimus dorsi muscles ("lats").

READY

Stand with your feet a few inches apart, holding a dumbbell in each hand.

SET

Raise both arms up so that the dumbbells are held about three inches higher than the top of your head, palms facing away from you. Spread your arms apart so that your arms form two 120-degree angles. If you look in the mirror, you should be able to see your lats clearly in this position. Your arms will be almost in the position people take when they are doing a double biceps pose, only slightly higher.

GO

Flex your lats as hard as possible and, keeping your elbows slightly to the front of you, lower the dumbbells until they reach just about ear height. Apply dynamic tension to your lat muscles as you return to start position, and repeat the movement until you have finished your set. Complete your final two sets, shake out your arms, and immediately move to the next exercise.

ATTENTION

It is crucial that you keep your mind riveted on your latissimus dorsi muscles throughout the exercise.

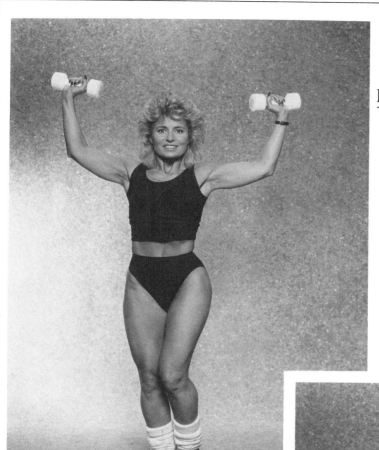

ID DUMBBELL LAT PULLDOWN
START

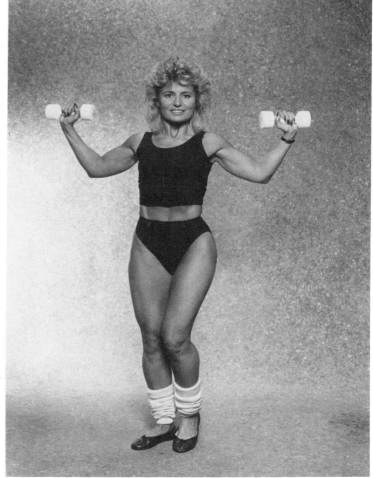

ID DUMBBELL LAT PULLDOWN
FINISH

ID DUMBBELL PREACHER CURLS– BICEPS EXERCISE #1
("PREACHERS")

Develops: Entire biceps muscle.

READY

Stand behind a chair with a dumbbell in your right hand.

SET

Tilt the chair backward and bend down until you are leaning on the floor with your left knee. Hold on to the chair with your left hand and place your right elbow on the back of the tilted chair. (The dumbbell is held in your right hand, palm facing upward.) You now have constructed a makeshift "preacher curl" bench.

GO

Controlling the tilt of the chair with your left hand, flex your right biceps as hard as possible with wrist locked and slightly bent toward you; as you apply isometric pressure, curl the dumbbell up until it grazes your nose. Apply dynamic tension as you return to start position, and repeat the movement until you have finished your set. Perform the exercise for the other arm, and continue to alternate back and forth until you have completed all three sets. Shake out your arms and immediately move to the next exercise.

ATTENTION

This exercise provides total isolation for your biceps muscle.

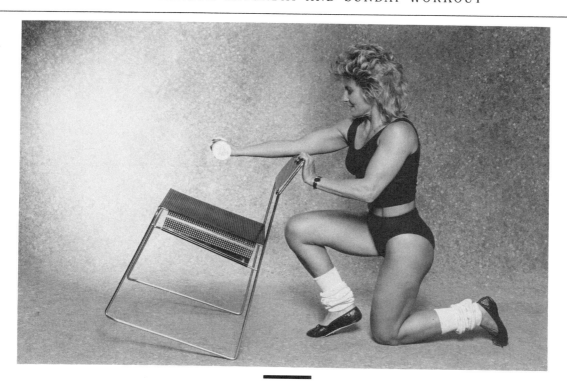

ID DUMBBELL PREACHER CURL
START

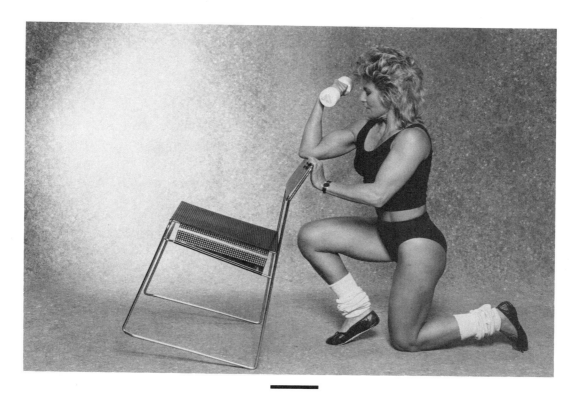

ID DUMBBELL PREACHER CURL
FINISH

Standing Simultaneous ID Dumbbell Curls—Biceps Exercise #2

("Simultaneous Curls")

Develops: The entire biceps area.

READY

Stand with your feet together or a few inches apart, holding a dumbbell in each hand.

SET

Hold the dumbbells with your palms facing away from you and your arms straight down at your sides. Keep your elbows and upper arms close to your body.

GO

Flex your biceps as hard as possible and, applying isometric pressure, simultaneously curl the dumbbells upward until you cannot curl any higher. Apply dynamic tension as you lower your arms to start position, and repeat the movement until you have finished your set. Complete your final two sets, shake out your arms, and immediately move to the next exercise.

ATTENTION

Look at your biceps muscle as it contracts as you apply isometric pressure and expands as you apply dynamic tension. Mentally picture it growing denser and more shapely.

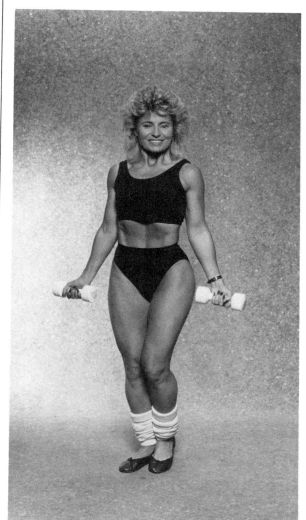

STANDING SIMULTANEOUS ID DUMBBELL CURL
START

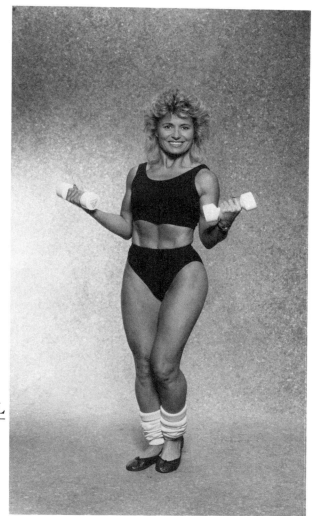

STANDING SIMULTANEOUS ID DUMBBELL CURL
FINISH

STANDING ONE-LEG ID DUMBBELL CALF RAISES— CALF EXERCISE #1

("STANDING RAISES")

Develops: The calf (gastrocnemius) muscle.

READY

Place a telephone directory, thick book, or attaché case on the floor near a chair.

SET

Hold a dumbbell with your left hand and stand on the book so that your heel and arch are completely off the book. (Note: The book should be high enough so that, when you extend your heel downward, your heel just about grazes the floor or doesn't touch it at all.) Raise your right foot off the floor so that it is out of the way and lower your left heel as low as possible.

GO

Apply isometric pressure to your left calf, flexing it as hard as possible and raise yourself up onto your toes. Apply the full force of dynamic tension as you return to start position, and repeat the movement until you have finished your set. Perform the set for your other leg, and continue to alternate legs until you have completed all three sets. Shake out your calves and jump for joy. Congratulations. You have completed your day six 12-minute workout, and you have worked your entire body twice in one week.

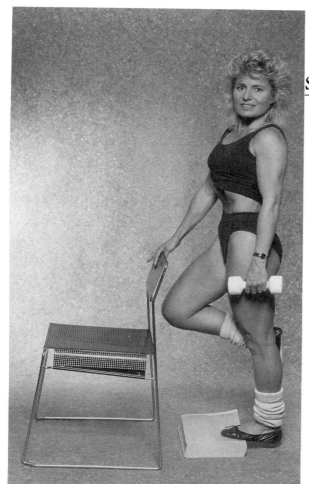

STANDING ONE-LEG ID DUMBBELL CALF RAISE
START

STANDING ONE-LEG ID DUMBBELL CALF RAISE
FINISH

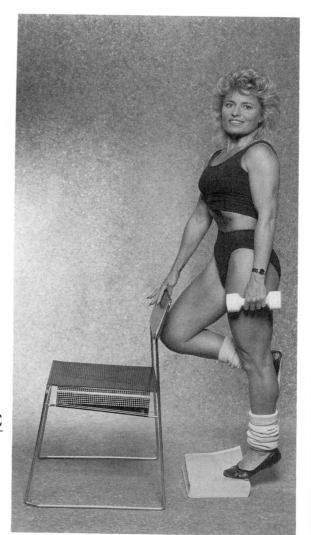

WORKOUT DAY SEVEN

Today is a relaxing day. All you have to do is work on your buttocks and abdominals in order to accomplish your necessary third weekly session. (You will recall that buttocks and abdominals need one extra weekly session in order to achieve perfect form. See page 33 for details.)

You may select any two buttocks exercises and any two abdominal exercises for your workout today. It's a good idea to pick one upper abdominal exercise and one lower abdominal exercise. You can do from 10 to 25 repetitions for each exercise. (Since this is a light day, you might want to take advantage of it and do the extra reps.) Buttocks exercises are found on pages 60-62 and 100-102. Abdominal exercises are found on pages 64-66 and 105-107. Soon you will have your entire routine memorized and will not have to refer to the book at all—except to remind you about form and isometric pressure and dynamic tension.

For your convenience, an exercise summary sheet is provided at the end of this chapter.

EXERCISE SUMMARY SHEET

MONDAY

CHEST: Flat ID dumbbell presses ("presses")

Incline ID dumbbell flyes ("flyes")

SHOULDERS: Front ID lateral raises ("front raises")

Pee-wee ID rear lateral raises ("pee-wee laterals")

TRICEPS: Double-arm ID kickbacks ("kickbacks")

Double-arm ID overhead extensions ("extensions")

TUESDAY

THIGHS: Fingertip ID squats ("squats")

Dumbbell ID lunges ("lunges")

BUTTOCKS: Dumbbell ID standing squeezes ("standing butt squeezes")

Kneeling ID angled leg lifts ("angled lifts")

ABDOMINALS: Dumbbell ID sit-ups ("sit-ups")

Dumbbell ID leg raises ("leg raises")

WEDNESDAY

BACK: Seated ID back laterals ("back laterals")

Standing ID leaning pulls ("leaning pulls")

BICEPS: Seated alternating ID dumbbell curls ("alternate curls")

Leaning ID concentration curls ("concentrations")

CALVES: Seated ID calf raises ("seated raises")

THURSDAY

CHEST: Standing ID dumbbell crossovers ("crossovers")

Seated ID dumbbell chest squeezes ("pec squeezes")

SHOULDERS: Standing ID side lateral raises ("side laterals")

Bent-over ID lateral raises ("bent laterals")

TRICEPS: Kneeling ID dumbbell pulldowns ("kneeling triceps pulldowns")

Standing ID dumbbell pushdowns ("pushdowns")

FRIDAY

THIGHS: Seated ID leg extensions ("extensions")

Lying ID leg curls ("leg curls")

BUTTOCKS: Seated ID scissors ("scissors")

Kneeling ID feather kick-ups ("feathers")

ABDOMINALS: Seated ID leg-ins ("leg-ins")

ID crunch twists ("crunch twists")

SATURDAY

BACK: Bent ID dumbbell rows ("bent rows")

ID dumbbell lat pulldowns ("lat pulldowns")

BICEPS: ID dumbbell preacher curls ("preachers")

Standing simultaneous ID dumbbell curls ("simultaneous curls")

CALVES: Standing one-leg ID dumbbell calf raises ("standing raises")

SUNDAY

BUTTOCKS: Any two buttocks exercises listed above.

ABDOMINALS: Any two abdominal exercises listed above.

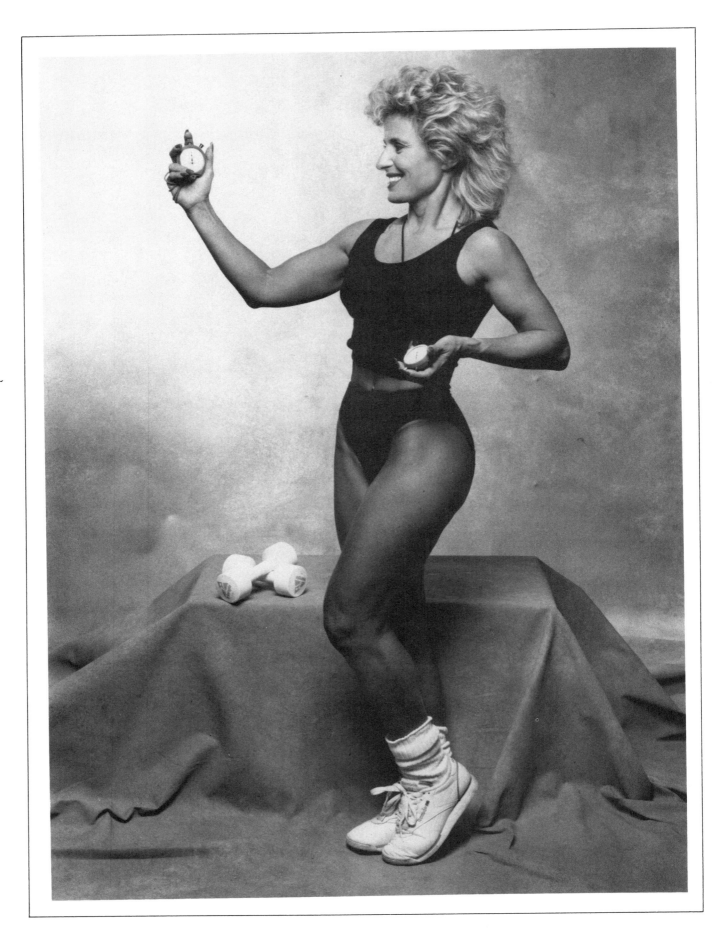

10

BURNING IT UP DOUBLE TIME

This chapter is for everyone who wants to see results "yesterday." We'll start with easy and go on to extremely difficult and arduous.

In order to speed up your progress and to perfect your overall body tone, there are certain things that are "musts" and certain things that are only for the fanatics. First the musts, then the fanatics.

"MUSTS" FOR PERFECTING THE BODY IN RECORD TIME

AEROBICS

An aerobic activity is one that causes the pulse rate to accelerate to between 70 and 80 percent of maximum capacity for a minimum of 20 minutes. (As noted earlier, your maximum pulse rate is calculated by subtracting your age from 220.)

Many people foolishly believe that aerobics can reshape the body. If this is so, why aren't runners the most esthetic of all athletes? No one would argue against that, in general, gymnasts, dancers, and martial artists have physiques that are much more appealing. Given this fact, why do I perform three 20- to 30-minute aerobic sessions per week? Why does anyone bother to do aerobics?

We do it because aerobic exercises serve a triple purpose: (1) They help to burn unwanted, unsightly body fat. (2) They help to strengthen the heart and lungs. (A stronger heart and lungs will enable you to perform your daily 12-minute routine more efficiently—and without heavy breathing.) (3) They help to increase blood circulation, which improves skin tone and causes one to look healthy—and, in effect, younger.

HOW MUCH AEROBICS SHOULD YOU DO?

In order to get the full benefit of an aerobic activity, you'll have to perform the exercise a minimum of three times a week for 20 minutes. For fitness purposes, your absolute maximum should be five 30-minute sessions. I do the minimum because I found out that more than that is a waste of my energy. I used to run five times a week for 30 minutes, and I didn't look any better than I do now. In fact, I think the additional aerobics actually helped to detract from my overall appearance, because I did not have too much additional body fat to get rid of, so the aerobics worked to tear down some of the hard-earned muscle I had built. Years of experimentation have taught me what I have to do to look my absolute best. I don't have time to invest one minute more than I have to in working out. I'm at the point in my life now where I don't work out just for the fun of it. I do it because I like the results—the way it makes me look and the way it makes me feel. If you are more than 10 pounds overweight, however, and want to get rid of fat as fast as possible, you can do the maximum amount of aerobics until you are less than 10 pounds overweight. After that, reduce to the minimum.

WHICH AEROBIC ACTIVITIES ARE BEST?

What's best is what's best for you. I hate the water. I'm a lion by nature (Leo) and I like to be on land. I also hate aerobic dancing because I'm somewhat of a klutz. I never feel as if I'm doing all the jumps and turns with grace and style. For this reason, I enjoy either running, walking fast, jumping rope, riding the stationary bicycle, or jumping on a trampoline. When I'm in California, I enjoy riding a bicycle or roller skating along the beach.

If you prefer to walk at a brisk pace, you can do so in place of the aerobic activity—but you'll have to double your time in order to get the same fast-burning effect. You won't get quite the same heart-lung stimulation since your pulse rate will not be accelerated as much, but don't worry about that. You'll get about 75 percent of the value, and that's fine. So if you choose to walk, you can walk for 40 minutes three times a week.

No matter which aerobic activity you choose, unless you're already conditioned to that activity, break in slowly. Start out with five minutes per session for the first week. Then go to 10 minutes per session the second week. Keep it at 10 minutes for two weeks, then go up to 15 minutes and remain there for two weeks. Now, after five weeks, you should be able to do a full 20 minutes. There are no hard and fast rules. It may take your body longer to get used to the aerobic activity.

Tune in to your body. Don't rush it. If you do, you may become disgusted and abandon the effort. Since fitness is going to become a lifetime habit for you, there's no need to drive yourself so hard in the beginning. If you ease into the program, and have respect for your body rather than abuse it, you'll find yourself feeling as if you're not paying a very high price to stay fit for the rest of your life.

WHEN IS THE BEST TIME TO PERFORM AEROBIC ACTIVITIES?

For me it's the morning. If I don't do it then, I don't want to do it later—and if I do, I look at it as a terrible punishment. Some people have told me they enjoy an aerobic session immediately after a long day of work. They claim it helps them to get rid of the tension of the workday. Others say they like to run or bicycle or do aerobic dancing during their lunch hour. They say that it's a perfect way to prevent themselves from eating a fattening lunch. Some even run just before going to bed. They claim it relaxes them. Experiment. If you fit exercise into your lifestyle with respect for your personality needs, it won't become the bane of your life. Instead you'll enjoy it.

EXERCISE SPURTS FROM NINE TO FIVE

I've often heard people brag, "I did my exercise this morning. Now I can vegetate for the rest of the day." This is not a very efficient or healthy way to stay in shape. It's better to exercise three or four times during the day in shorter spurts than to exercise, say, for a full hour in the morning and then do nothing else all day. Person A exercises in the morning, and then stagnates all day. Her metabolism speeds up for about an hour after the exercise, then returns to its normal level and remains that way all day. Person B exercises for 12 minutes in the morning and then three times during the day for approximate 12-minute spurts. Her metabolism speeds up each of the four times she exercises, and remains accelerated for about an hour each time she does so. Person B has burned more calories than person A, even though person B has actually exercised less in actual minutes. For example, say person A and person B each consumed 1,800 calories, and all other things such as body weight, general activity, and general basal metabolism are the same. Person A would burn up about 1,800 calories, but person B would burn about 2,100.

Here are some suggestions for exercise spurts. They can be performed whether you work out of your home or in an office.

Take a short walk before and/or after lunch. There are many ways to do this. The most convenient way is to select a restaurant that is 12 minutes' walking distance from your place of business. This way you'll get the double benefit of a walk before and after lunch. If not, you could take a 12-minute walk and then go to lunch. If you work at home, what's stopping you from going outside and taking a brisk walk before lunch or after lunch? (If you have to choose, it's a better idea to walk right after lunch. This will ensure the most efficient burning of calories if your goal is to lose excess fat.)

Jumping-jack breaks. Some time between lunch and going home, take a 12-minute break and do jumping jacks. You can do this in the lounge or restroom if there's no other convenient place. Take off your suit jacket and blouse and throw on a T-shirt. Remove your shoes and jump. You'll be just about starting to sweat when you stop. If anyone comes in and sees you, they'll think you're crazy at first, but don't worry. After their initial shock, they'll probably be thinking about how they wish they had your discipline. If you work at home, you may find it relaxing to take a short, 12-minute jumping-jack break. You may be surprised to find that you approach the job at hand with renewed vigor.

Walking to and from work. If you drive to work, park 12 minutes away and walk. This will enable you to do two exercise spurts per day—one going to work and another going home. If you think you'll need your car during the workday, so what? You can still park 12 minutes away, then walk to your car when you need it. Then when you return to work, you can park close by. If you take a train or bus to work, you can get off a few stops before your usual stop and walk. If you could walk the entire distance in 45 minutes or less, why not forget transportation and walk it? I do this whenever I'm in Manhattan and I have to take care of business in various parts of town. I'll wear a pair of Reeboks and carry my heels in my briefcase. Some days I'll walk at least 45 minutes. If you choose to walk to work, you probably won't lose any time, since traffic and/or waiting for buses and trains often consume the same amount of time it would take to walk.

Walking up stairs. Make up your mind to give up escalators completely, and to use elevators only when there are more than six floors to walk. True, your stair walking won't take 12 minutes, but added up over time, it will help your fitness program considerably.

Stand rather than sit. Don't throw this book across the room yet. I'm not asking you to work on your feet all day. But if you do ride a bus or the subway, why not stand on the way to work if your job is one that requires you to sit all day? And why not stand on the way home, too? After all, when you get home, you'll be sitting again. "But my feet hurt," you say. Ridiculous. I can't believe you're still wearing painful high heels to work and not comfortable soft-cushioned aerobic or tennis shoes.

Once you are at work, instead of sitting all day long while you do your work, make it your business to stand up for 12 minutes at a time once in a while. You can still do the work you would ordinarily do sitting. Get in the habit of standing while you're on the telephone, for example. I'll bet you could think of 10 others things you could do standing instead of sitting.

ESPECIALLY FOR THE HARDEST WORKERS OF ALL: FULL-TIME HOUSEWIVES AND MOTHERS

You can incorporate all of the above into your own lifestyle. Instead of walking to or from work, you can take a brief, brisk walk every morning. It would be worth your while to do so early in the morning, if necessary—before your husband or an older child leaves the house, if you have toddlers who can't be left alone. If this is impossible, make it your business to take a brisk walk during the day with your toddler. Pushing a stroller or baby carriage while walking at a brisk pace will provide even more exercise. I used to do that when my daughter was a baby, and it really helped to keep me in shape. You may not feel like going out and walking, but once you're on the move, you'll be glad you did it. You'll feel energized and refreshed because you will have stimulated your entire body. Many people don't realize that walking is one of the best overall body toners, so the more walking you can fit into your busy day, the better.

LET'S NOT GO OVERBOARD

By now you may be thinking that this whole thing is going to become a burden to you, so you'd just as well forget the whole program. Of course I don't want you to become so obsessed with these suggestions that you feel guilty every time you sit down or park near work or take an escalator. I suggest that instead you pick out any three of the above suggestions and incorporate them into your daily life. Forget the rest.

ACCELERATING THE 12-MINUTE WORKOUT

You can intensify and accelerate your daily 12-minute workout by "supersetting," or "giant-setting." These methods are not "musts" for accelerating your progress. They're options, and they may help to make the routine less boring after you have been working out for about three months. (Please don't try them before that time, because I want you to become totally accustomed to the movements of the workout so you do not sacrifice form for speed.)

There are two ways to superset: (1) supersetting within a given body part; (2) supersetting while working two different body parts.

SUPERSETTING WITHIN A GIVEN BODY PART

You can superset any body part. Let's use the shoulders as an example.

In your Monday shoulder routine, you are required to do two exercises, front raises and pee-wee laterals. To superset these two exercises, do your first set of front raises and, without resting, do your first set of pee-wee laterals. Then take a 10-second rest. Next, do your second set of front raises and pee-wee laterals and take another 10-second rest. Finally, do your third superset of raises and pee-wee laterals. You will have completed your three supersets and you will have finished your shoulder routine—and in record time, because you will have eliminated some rest periods. But what's more important, you will have intensified your workout. You can superset all three body parts on a given day. For example, your Monday routine consists of chest, shoulders, and triceps. You could superset your chest exercises, alternating presses and flyes; your shoulder exercises, alternating raises and pee-wee laterals (as described above); and your triceps, alternating kickbacks and extensions. You will then have supersetted your entire Monday workout of chest, shoulders, and triceps.

SUPERSETTING WHEN WORKING TWO DIFFERENT BODY PARTS

You can superset any two body parts on a given day. Let's use the Monday routine again as an example. On that day you will be exercising chest, shoulders, and triceps. You can superset chest with shoulders, for example. Do your first set of presses for your chest and, without resting, continue with your first set of raises for your shoulders. Rest 10 seconds and then perform your second set of presses and raises. Then rest 10 seconds again and perform your final superset of presses and raises. You will then have completed a superset for your first exercise of both your chest and shoulder routines. But there are two exercises in each routine, so you will now have to superset your second exercise in each of these body part routines. You will superset your flyes (your chest exercise) with your pee-wee laterals (your shoulder exercise). Now you will have completed supersets working out the two body parts for the entire routine.

GIANT-SETTING

A giant set is really a bigger superset. Instead of doing two exercises at a time, you do three. This workout lends itself very neatly to giant sets among body parts, since you exercise three body parts each day, except Sundays. (In this workout, it is not possible to giant-set within a body part, since only two exercises are required for each body part on a given day, and three exercises are needed in order to giant-set.) Let's use the Monday workout as an example again. Your Monday routine consists of chest, shoulders, and triceps. Do the first set of your chest exercise, presses; the first set of your shoulder exercise, raises; and the first set of your triceps exercise, kickbacks. Then rest 10 seconds and perform the second set for each of the above exercises. Rest 10 seconds and complete the final set for each of the above exercises. Then rest about 20 seconds and proceed to giant-set the second exercise for each body part. Do the first set of flyes for your chest, the first set of pee-wee laterals for your shoulders, and the first set of extensions for your triceps. Then rest 10 seconds and complete the second set for each of the above exercises. Again, rest 10 seconds and complete the final set for each of the above exercises. You will have giant-setted the entire Monday workout: chest, shoulders, and triceps. You can giant-set any day's workout (except Sunday, of course, because there are only two body parts being exercised on Sunday and a giant set requires three exercises).

PERFECTING TROUBLESOME BODY PARTS

If you have a body part that you want really to attack, do the exercises for that body part two additional times during the week. For example, suppose you want to do additional work on your thighs. If you usually do your 12-minute daily workout in the morning, do the additional thigh workout at night. It's a good idea to leave one day between workouts for a given body part, however. So, since thighs are exercised on Tuesdays and Fridays, you can work them additionally on Wednesday night and Sunday night.

You should use the above system for any troublesome body part, but if your problem areas are buttocks or abdominals, you don't have to worry about leaving a day's rest between workouts. These body parts respond well to daily workouts. If you wish, you can work them four days in a row or even six days a week. (One day of rest for a body part, no matter how troublesome, is a good idea. It prevents burnout.)

FOR FANATICS ONLY

If you're in a mad rush to get into shape, you could do the 12-minute workout twice a day. You would do Monday's workout Monday morning, Tuesday's workout Monday night, and Wednesday's workout Tuesday morning and Thursday's workout Tuesday night, and so on. By the middle of the week you will have completed the week's workout, but you will not stop there. You'll begin with Monday again, so that by the end of the week, you will have completed the workout twice instead of once, and you will have worked all of your body parts four times that week instead of two times (except buttocks and abdominals, which you will have worked six times that week instead of three times). Frankly, I don't recommend working out twice a day this way unless you're very highly motivated. It's an awful lot of work and you may rebel against the entire program. But you know yourself better than I do. If you're the type of person who wants to see results quickly and is willing to pay the price, try it. But after you begin to see progress (in about three weeks) switch to the once-daily routine or burnout is just around the corner. I would never do this twice a day. The mere thought of it exhausts me.

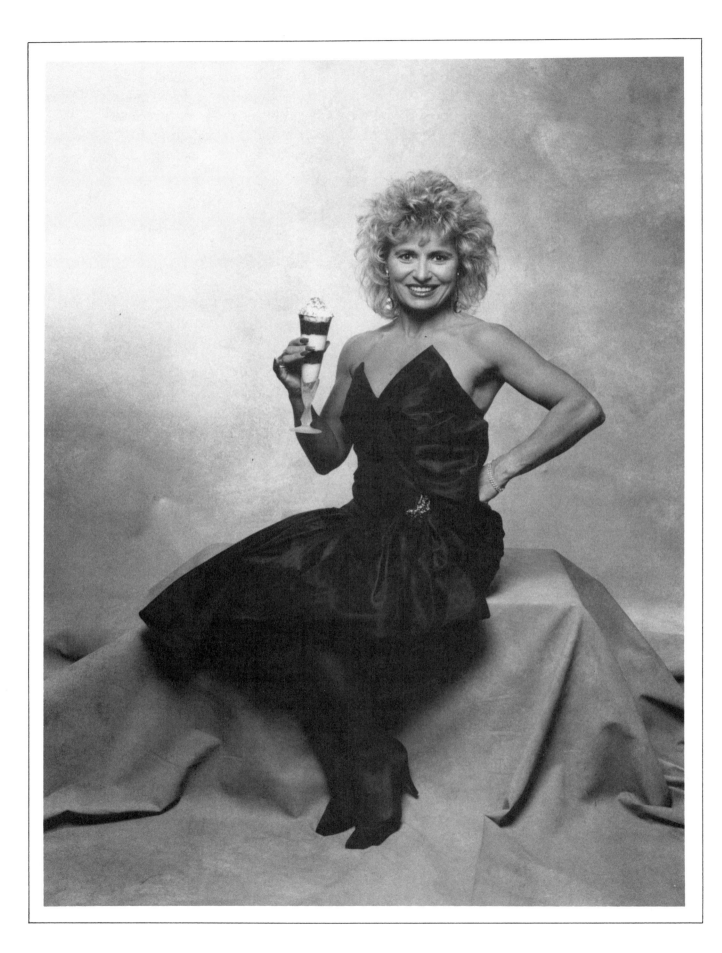

11

MAKING FRIENDS WITH FOOD

Food is not an enemy. If that's true, why do most of us feel guilty every time we put something in our mouths? This unnecessary burden of guilt is the result of ignorance and its bedfellow, fear. When we don't know how something works, we can't control it—so we usually fear it.

I used to live in fear of food. I would starve myself all day long and eat one big meal every night. When that didn't work to get me in shape, I started running five miles a day. But despite all my efforts, except for my calves, my body was soft and out of shape, and I was overweight. It got to the point that whenever I ate anything at all, I felt guilty. I began thinking, Something is wrong. We need food to stay alive. It should be a normal, enjoyable part of life. I decided to do something about my problem.

Determined to learn the basic rules of good nutrition, I began interviewing the athletes who, in my opinion, had the leanest looking, most muscular bodies—professional bodybuilders. That's when I learned that dieting, like any other body-related program, is an exact science. I dared to follow their advice and gave up my unproductive dieting. Instead of starving all day and eating only once a day, I now ate five times a day. To my amazement, I was never hungry the way I used to be, yet I lost excess fat-weight, because now I knew what to eat and when to eat it—and I didn't have to give up my favorite "goodies," either.

NEVER AGAIN WILL YOU FEAR FOOD

Most people have an "approach-avoidance" complex when it comes to food. Their mixed feelings remind one of the rats in an experiment performed some years ago by scientists. Rats were kept in a cage where food was stored just behind a grid that, when touched, produced an electric shock. Every time the rats lunged for the food, they were greeted by a painful electrical charge. As a result, whenever the rats would think of food, they experienced mixed emotions—they would look forward to eating with joy, but at the same time they would tremble and hesitate in fear of the electric shock. Such mixed emotions have come to be known as "approach-avoidance" feelings.

The goal of this chapter is to free you from approach-avoidance feelings toward food, and to help you to understand how food works to build and nourish your body. You will be in control. Guilt and fear will become a thing of the past, even when you eat your most "sinful" foods, such as chocolate, doughnuts, ice-cream, cake, or even fast foods. In fact, you can regularly indulge in your favorite food treats once you know what you're doing.

WHAT ARE CALORIES AND WILL YOU HAVE TO COUNT THEM?

THE ENERGY IN A CALORIE

A calorie is a unit of chemical energy released to your body every time the food you eat is digested. Most active women need between 2,000 and 2,300 calories to maintain their normal weight, and women who do no exercise at all need at least 1,200 to 1,500. (If you are following this exercise program, consider yourself an active woman.)

CALORIES BURNED IN VARIOUS ACTIVITIES

As long as you're alive, you're burning calories. You burn about 40 calories an hour just breathing—when you are in a state of total rest, such as sitting in a chair or sleeping. So, even if you were in a coma and slept all day, you would have to be fed at least 880 calories a day to maintain your body weight. Even the most sedentary person uses more energy than that. Energy is expended when we take showers, brush our teeth, talk on the telephone, drive a car, or even read a book.

You can see, then, how any "work" helps to burn calories. For example, a brisk 12-minute walk burns about 80 calories, while a 12-minute run burns double that amount. The 12-Minute Daily Workout burns about 100 calories, and walking up and down stairs for 12 minutes burns about 120 calories. Swimming at an easy pace for 12 minutes burns about 100 calories, doing jumping jacks for 12 minutes burns about 150 calories, and riding a bicycle at a brisk pace for 12 minutes burns about 75 calories. Doing these short exercises can burn at least 250 additional calories a day.

CALORIES IN SPECIFIC FOODS

Food is made up of three major elements: fat, carbohydrate, and protein. Fat yields 9 calories per gram, but carbohydrates and protein yield only 4 calories per gram. Obviously, fat is the least desirable of food sources if you are seeking to lose weight—or your own fat. But fat is an undesirable food source for yet another reason.

SOME CALORIES ARE "FATTER" THAN OTHERS

When you consume carbohydrates or protein, your body has to do a certain amount of work in order to metabolize those calories—and it burns up some calories during this digestive process. Fat, on the other hand, can be deposited directly in adipose storage cells overlying your muscle tissue—almost no calories are expended in digesting the fat. As it turns out, that semiserious remark about that pint of ice-cream going straight to your hips is true. What was once believed to be fact—that all calories are of equal value—has proven to be a myth. The fact is, if you were to consume 2,000 calories in fat alone, you would gain more weight than someone who consumed 2,000 calories in protein and carbohydrates.

CALORIE AWARENESS RATHER THAN CALORIE COUNTING

In order to lose one pound of fat, you must create an approximate 3,500-calorie deficit in your body. But I don't want you to count calories. I want you instead to become aware of calories by developing a feel for them. In reading this chapter, your mind, which is somewhat like a highly sophisticated computer, will register the facts about calories. After this, whenever you approach food with the thought of possibly eating it, you will begin automatically to calculate its desirability in terms of caloric value. To assist your mind in its job, I suggest that you purchase one of the nutrition books listed in the bibliography, and browse through the lists of food content at your leisure. What you read in that book, in combination with the information in this chapter, will enable you to automatically discriminate among foods whenever you eat—you will not have to take out a calculator to verify nutritional value; you will know what's good for you and what's not.

FAT

So far we've discussed the negative aspects of fat, but fat has some positive qualities as well. Your body needs a certain amount of fat in order to be healthy. About 15 to 18 percent of your food intake should be fat. Most people consume much more than that—some as high as 45 to 50 percent. Small wonder so many people are themselves fat. If someone were totally deprived of fat, however, that person would be unable to absorb vitamins A, E, K, and D and the mineral calcium. That person's internal organs would have no cushion and would possibly be damaged by the slightest sudden movement.

WHY DO WE GET FAT?

Getting fat is a biological survival strategy. When you consume excess fat, it is stored under the skin for possible future use. The body is not vain. It does not care that the additional adipose tissue covers your shapely muscles and makes you look like a butterball. Unaware that you live in a country where food is plentiful, when you overeat your body takes advantage of the opportunity to hoard the extra food as fat, saving it to use as fuel (energy) in case there is a future famine.

SOURCES OF FAT

You'll never have to worry about not getting enough fat in your diet. Even if you totally avoid "fat demons" such as fried foods, ice-cream, full-fat milk and milk products, red meats, etc., your diet will contain at least 18 percent fat. You'll get most of your fat when you eat proteins. Even white-meat chicken, a well-known low-fat source of protein, has a certain amount of fat. For example, eight ounces of skinned chicken contains about 10 grams, or 90 calories, of fat. (The other calories in the chicken are protein—about 70 grams, or 280 calories.) So of the 370 calories in the chicken, one-fourth will have been fat. Even low-fat fish such as flounder contains some fat. Believe it or not, natural carbohydrate foods also contain small amounts of fat. An apple has one-half gram or 4 calories of fat, and so does a cup of spinach. (Check *The Nutrition Almanac* for details.)

You can see, then, that no matter how strict your diet, you will be getting enough fat to fulfill the minimum requirement. You'll have to wait until you've reached your weight goal before you can indulge in fried foods, ice-cream, red meat, and other fatty foods, and even then you'll have to limit them to once a week.

FIBER IN THE DIET HELPS TO ELIMINATE FAT

When fiber is consumed, since it cannot be digested, it passes through your system unregistered as stored energy—and it takes with it about 10 percent of the fat found in your digestive tract at the time it passes through. If you get plenty of fiber in your diet, you will automatically eliminate 10 percent of the fat you eat before it registers on your body as fat. (There are other reasons for getting lots of fiber in your diet. See Complex Carbohydrates, pages 141 and 145, for further information.)

CHOLESTEROL

Cholesterol is "saturated" fat—animal fat in hard form—as opposed to "unsaturated"—vegetable, nut, or grain fat in liquid form. In spite of its bad reputation, a certain amount of cholesterol is beneficial to your health. Cholesterol converts to vitamin D in sunlight, and it helps you to digest carbohydrates. It also helps to form cortisone and sex hormones. But too much cholesterol causes arteriosclerosis and heart attacks. If you think your cholesterol level is too high, get a cholesterol count. In the meantime, eat eggplant, onions, yogurt, apples, soybeans, pinto beans, and kidney beans. Avoid excessive caffeine, refined sugar, saturated fats, and, by all means, stop smoking.

Not too long ago, the egg was attacked as a dangerous cholesterol-producing enemy. But recent research has proven that in fact the nutrients in eggs help to *break up cholesterol deposits,* and carry them away from the blood vessel walls to the liver for excretion. Eggs do this by helping to raise beneficial HDL (high-density lipoprotein) levels.

CARBOHYDRATES

Carbohydrates are the body's main source of energy. The moment you eat a carbohydrate, your body begins breaking it down into glucose, or "blood sugar." Without glucose, you wouldn't be able to think clearly. Your central nervous system would slow down to a grinding halt, and you'd become sluggish and irritable. Your body would go into an "emergency" mode of operation and would begin converting protein and then muscle tissue into glucose. In other words, your body would begin "eating itself." This is why high-protein/low-carbohydrate diets are self-defeating. When denied carbohydrates, the body loses water (because carbohydrates hold water) and begins eating muscle tissue. Fat remains intact. Your body weight goes down because of water and muscle loss, and once you stop the diet, your overall body composition is higher in fat than before, so it is softer and flabbier than ever—and your weight goes up again as soon as you regain the lost water and start building more fat again.

About two-thirds of your calorie consumption should consist of carbohydrates. There are three types of carbohydrates: processed, simple, and complex.

PROCESSED CARBOHYDRATES

These are sugars in every form—sucrose (table sugar), glucose, dextrose, maltose, lactose, fructose, sorbitol, and xylitol. If you see any of these names on a label, realize that you are about to consume sugar with a fancy name. Bleached flour is also a processed carbohydrate. Processed carbohydrates are undesirable sources of energy because they raise your blood sugar level too quickly. They give you a spurt of energy, but about 20 minutes later your blood sugar level drops to *below* its initial level, producing an immediate craving for more sugar. You are compelled to consume more and more sugar in order to keep your energy level up. In the end, you consume many empty calories, and you gain weight.

SIMPLE CARBOHYDRATES

These are carbohydrates found in all fruits. When you eat a piece of fruit, the carbohydrates go straight to your bloodstream and you get an immediate shot of energy. But with simple carbohydrates, as opposed to processed carbohydrates, you don't pay the price of an energy deficit 20 minutes later, and you are not compelled to go back for more.

COMPLEX CARBOHYDRATES

Vegetables, grains, and pasta are complex carbohydrates. The prolonged enzymatic action of these carbohydrates as they are broken down into simple sugars produces a gradually released supply of energy. For this reason, they are even more valuable than simple carbohydrates, which supply immediate but shorter-lived energy.

COMPLEX CARBOHYDRATES AND FIBER

Whole grains, fruits, and vegetables are the only foods that contain *dietary fiber*. Most people have a vague idea about the importance of fiber in the diet. They believe (and rightly so) that fiber helps to prevent cancer and that it aids in the elimination process—so they make noble attempts to increase fiber in their diet by religiously downing a spoon or two of wheat germ or eating whole-wheat bread instead of white bread.

In addition to the fact that fiber helps to eliminate fat from your system, it provides yet another benefit—some "free calories." Here's how it works: When calories are calculated for a given complex carbohydrate, the calories of the fiber content of that food are included in the calculation. But the body is incapable of digesting fiber because our intestines lack the enzymes required to break down these rough substances. Since most complex carbohydrates consist of about 10 percent fiber, you actually get 10 percent worth of free calories when you consume a complex carbohydrate—a real food bargain for those who are seeking to eat as much as they can without getting fat.

PROTEIN

The major component of your muscles, hair, nails, blood, and internal organs is protein, and it's protein that helps to regulate the water balance and the metabolism of your body.

Protein consists of 22 elements known as "amino acids." The human body can produce 14 of these, but in order to obtain the other eight we must eat foods that contain them. These foods include: red meat, poultry, eggs, fish, milk, and milk products. About 15 to 18 percent of the diet should consist of protein.

A WORD ABOUT VITAMINS AND MINERALS

Vitamins and minerals in the right combination are necessary for good health. Vitamins, such as A, B-complex, B-1, B-2, B-6, B-12, C, D, E, and niacin, are organic substances found in green and yellow vegetables, meat, fish, poultry, rice, and other whole grains. Minerals such as iron, magnesium, phosphorus, potassium, sodium, and calcium are nutrients found in organic and inorganic combinations in foods such as green vegetables, beef, organ meats, fish, poultry, whole grains, and fruit. If you remember to eat plenty of green and yellow vegetables, and you do not neglect fish, chicken, organ meats, and whole grains, your diet will not lack sufficient vitamins and minerals. However, if you want to analyze your particular diet, see the bibliography for a special vitamin book to help you do so.

CALCIUM

The mineral calcium is worthy of special attention, because calcium deficiency causes thinning and weakening bones. Women and men are most susceptible to this condition after the age of 30.

Other than proper diet, the best way to ensure against thinning bones is regularly to do weight-bearing exercises (such as the ones described in this book). Patricia Hausman, M.S., author of *The Calcium Bible*, says, "Bone experts believe that to build bone, you have to exercise the area of the body in which you want improvement to occur. To strengthen your wrist, for instance, researchers believe that you must work this area directly..."[1] As you have seen, *The 12-Minute Total-Body Workout* exercises *each* body part at least two times a week!

The United States government recommends a minimum of 800 to 1,200 milligrams of calcium daily; however, most doctors feel that to be on the safe side, 1,500 milligrams should be consumed daily. Each of the following foods in the quantities described contains 100 milligrams of calcium.

One cup skim milk

Two-thirds cup low-fat cottage cheese

Eight ounces plain yogurt

One-half cup low-fat ricotta cheese

One-half ounce American cheese

One cup farina

Two-thirds cup oatmeal

Two-thirds cup wheat cereal

One cup broccoli

One cup kale

One cup cooked soybeans

One cup collard greens

One cup turnip greens

Four ounces shrimp

Ten okra pods

The best source of calcium, or of any vitamin or mineral for that matter, is food, not food supplements. If you feel you're not getting enough calcium in your diet, consult your doctor and he will recommend the appropriate calcium supplement for your particular dietary needs.

WHAT ABOUT SODIUM, OR SALT?

A deficiency of the mineral sodium can result in muscle cramping. I've seen this happen to athletes who, in an effort to gain maximum definition of the muscles (a condition they call "ripped") for bodybuilding contests, have depleted their bodies of sodium. (The recommended daily sodium intake is betwen 1,500 and 2,500 milligrams. Some medical authorities differ slightly on either end of the scale.) These athletes often consume less than 500 milligrams of sodium each day for a week prior to a contest—a difficult task, since even a glass of tap water contains about 10 milligrams of sodium.

Because sodium helps to regulate body fluids, a deficiency causes dehydration, while an overabundance causes water retention. Sodium holds up to 50 times its own weight in water. If you consume a large bowl of canned soup, for example (containing 2,000 milligrams of sodium), and a cheeseburger with a pickle for dinner (another 2,000 milligrams of sodium), the next day you will weigh, look, and feel a few pounds fatter because of water retention.

If you don't have a problem with hypertension and you don't mind carrying around a few pounds of water bloat, however, you may want to do what I do in the winter. I love salty foods. I could eat a whole jar of pickles and live on canned soups and Chinese food for the rest of my life. I would trade a pint of my favorite ice-cream for a bagel-and-lox sandwich in a minute. Since I have very low blood pressure, I don't have to watch my sodium intake. I don't care if I look a few pounds fatter in the cold New York winter, when I'm not strolling on the beach in a two-piece bathing suit. I realize that I can shed the extra three or so pounds of water in a matter of five to seven days if I drop my sodium level to between 1,500 and 2,500 milligrams.

My purpose for telling you this is not to encourage you to follow in my footsteps, but to show you that you can indulge in high-sodium foods without gaining permanent weight—if you don't have high blood pressure, and if your doctor approves.

If you don't want to carry around an extra three pounds of water, however, consider this. Most people consume at least double the daily recommended amount of sodium. It's hidden in many foods. For example, two tablespoons of A-1 sauce contain 550 milligrams of sodium, a six-ounce slice of pizza 1,000 milligrams, and a medium-size frankfurter 840 milligrams.

There's plenty of sodium in fish, chicken, beef, and fresh fruits and vegetables. You don't have to go out of your way to get it. A lettuce and tomato salad with no dressing contains about 50 milligrams of sodium; a half cantaloupe, 25 milligrams; eight ounces of flounder, 800 milligrams; eight ounces of chicken breast, 150 milligrams; and eight ounces of ground round beef, 150 milligrams. You can see where it's possible to get your full minimum allotment of 1,500 milligrams of sodium without ever using table salt (2,000 milligrams per teaspoon).

WATER

It's appropriate to talk about water immediately after sodium because most people have a misconception about how the two elements work together.

People mistakenly believe that the more water they drink, the more they will retain. In fact, the opposite is true. Water flushes out your system. The more you drink, the more you eliminate—and with it, the toxins that might otherwise remain in your system. Drinking water is the only way to bathe the inside of your body. Think of it this way: Every time you drink a glass of plain water, you give your internal organs a shower.

Most of us don't drink enough water. Six to eight 8-ounce glasses of plain water (mineral, spring, or tap) a day is ideal. Try to drink a glass of water in the morning when you rise and at night before bedtime, and a glass before and after each meal. It isn't easy, but once you establish the habit you'll feel much better, and your skin will look younger, too. In addition, it helps to curb your appetite, especially that glass you drink before a meal.

REMINDERS:

Fat. The worst calories: (1) 9 calories per ounce as opposed to 4 calories per ounce for protein and carbohydrates. (2) Its calories are deposited directly in your tissue (go straight to your hips). (3) Fat costs you more in calories because nothing is burned up in the digestive process.

Processed Carbohydrates (sugars and bleached flours). These cause energy let-downs and encourage overeating.

Sodium. Excess sodium causes water retention, which makes you appear a few pounds fatter, but this excess water can be eliminated in five to seven days by dropping your sodium level.

Water. Drink lots of it to cleanse your system, curb your appetite, and have younger, healthier-looking skin.

Fiber. Eat lots of complex carbohydrates. Most contain at least 10 percent fiber—which results in 10 percent "free" calories.

DIET: IT DIDN'T TAKE TWO WEEKS TO GAIN THE WEIGHT

Most people go along enjoying life and food, while slowly gaining pounds of fat. Then something happens. Maybe they try on pants that fit perfectly a year ago, and can't get the zipper closed; perhaps they run into an old friend who asks, "Haven't you gained weight?" Or maybe, in a brave moment, they step on the scale, and see a 10-pound gain. At this point, they panic and say,

"I'm going to get rid of this weight if it kills me," and they demand to lose all of the excess weight in a week or two, when the fact is, it probably took months to gain.

Why does it seem as if it happened overnight? The simple truth is, you were under no pressure to gain weight, so you weren't monitoring yourself. You weren't thinking about it at all—were in fact busy dealing with your life. But, unbeknownst to you, you were gaining about half a pound a week. Even the notoriously fat man or woman you read about in the paper who weighs over 500 pounds didn't gain more than about a pound or two a week—50 to 100 pounds a year. (If you've seen a scale jump of more than a pound or two in a week, it was water retention. See the discussion on sodium, pages 143-145.)

YOU CAN LOSE WEIGHT FASTER THAN YOU GAINED IT

There's good news. You can actually lose weight faster than you gained it—only it will not seem that way because you will be aware of what you're doing when you're losing it. In other words, you'll be self-conscious. It's inevitable. You've heard the expression "A watched pot never boils." It may seem to you that it's taking forever to lose this weight. But in truth, you will lose it faster than you gained it. Chances are you didn't gain more than a pound and a half a week, or more than 70 to 80 pounds in a year. In fact, you probably didn't gain more than 30 pounds in a year. (That would be about half a pound a week.) But if you follow the diet and exercise program in this book, I can guarantee that you will lose at least a pound a week, and probably more—a pound and a half a week. And, what's more important, I can promise you that with the way of eating I'm going to show you, you'll keep the weight off. In addition, you'll be relieved, once and for all, of your fear of food and of the guilt you experience every time you eat your favorite fattening food.

WHY YOU WILL END UP FATTER IF YOU TRY TO LOSE MORE THAN A POUND AND A HALF A WEEK

The human body is incapable of losing much more than a pound and a half of fat a week. If you go on a starvation diet, your body will lose more than a pound and a half in weight, but a portion of that weight will be muscle tissue—the body will literally begin to eat itself. Then one day your survival instinct will take over when you're off guard, and you will stuff yourself with everything you've been missing. You will gain more weight than you lost on the diet. But that's not the worst part. When you come off a starvation diet (anything under 1,000 calories a day is dangerously close to starvation), the weight you gain back does not evenly redistribute itself into muscle weight and fat weight, even though you lost both muscle and fat—it goes back on your body as fat only. The body is incapable of storing excess food as muscle (only working out can prompt muscle growth). So the end result of your attempted shortcut is a fatter, more out-of-shape body than before you started the diet.

GENERAL RULES FOR LOSING WEIGHT AND HEALTHY DIETING

1. Your diet should consist of about 68 percent carbohydrates, 15 to 18 percent protein, and 15 to 18 percent fat. (You will automatically consume most of your fat requirement when you eat proteins, and a small amount when you eat carbohydrates. (See the discussion on fat for details.)

2. Reduce your caloric intake to from 1,500 to 1,800 calories a day. Eating less than 1,000 calories a day can reduce your metabolic rate. The American Dietetic Association recommends that you eat at least 10 calories per pound of body weight when you want to lose weight. I agree. You don't actually have to count calories, but you should become "calorie aware."

3. Avoid processed sugars.

4. Eat more complex carbohydrates than simple carbohydrates. (Remember, the roughage helps to eliminate 10 percent of the fat you consume before it is digested and registers on your body as fat.)

5. Avoid all fats and fatty foods until you have reached your goal weight (this includes ice-cream, red meat, the dark meat of poultry, full-fat milk and cheeses, and all fried foods).

6. Drink a glass of water before each meal and whenever you feel slightly hungry, *before* you have your snack. You won't feel like it. Force yourself to do it. You can put some lemon or an ounce of orange juice in the water, and you can drink it at room temperature—

it goes down easier that way. (As you might have guessed, I'm not in love with water.)

7. Limit your alcoholic beverages to two glasses of white wine or champagne per week. If possible, cut alcohol out altogether until you have reached goal weight.

WEIGHT-LOSS FOODS

If you stick to the following delicious foods, you'll have a great time losing your pound to pound and a half a week.

SIMPLE CARBOHYDRATES

All fruits except apricots, cranberries, currants, dates, figs, grapes, prunes, raisins, and watermelon. (These are excellent fruits for your maintenance diet once you have reached your weight goal.) Bananas are slightly high in calories, but you can have one or two a week without hurting your weight-loss program. Don't bore yourself to death with only apples, grapefruit, oranges, and cantaloupe. Try other fruits, such as blackberries, peaches, nectarines, pomegranates, raspberries, and rhubarb.

COMPLEX CARBOHYDRATES

The most calorie-economic and hunger-satisfying of the complex carbohydrates are the following: a large baked or boiled potato, two-thirds cup white or brown rice, four ounces high-protein or whole-wheat pasta, two-thirds cup oatmeal, two slices whole-wheat bread, two-thirds cup bran cereal, a small bran muffin, one ear of corn. Everything on the above list is about 100 calories—except the pasta, which is 200 calories.

Eat plenty of green, yellow, and red vegetables such as broccoli, carrots, celery, cucumbers, onions, peppers, spinach, tomatoes, and lettuce. Don't stick to the same old vegetables all the time. Push yourself to eat alfalfa sprouts, brussels sprouts, chard, chives, eggplant, endive, kale, leeks, mushrooms, mustard greens, pumpkin, radishes, rutabaga, scallions, shallots, turnips, turnip greens, and watercress.

PROTEIN

The most calorie-economic proteins are white-meat chicken and turkey, flounder, haddock, perch, shrimp, snapper, sole, tuna in water, eggs (the whites), low-fat cottage cheese, low-fat plain yogurt, and organ meats (kidney, liver, heart, etc.). After you've reached your weight goal, you can add limited portions of beef, bass, bluefish, carp, halibut, herring, mackerel, oysters, salmon, swordfish, trout, whitefish, and various cheeses.

FOR PEOPLE WHO COME HOME STARVING AND HAVE LITTLE PATIENCE OR TIME TO COOK

Stock your refrigerator with plenty of the above-listed fresh and frozen fruits and vegetables. (You can also purchase canned, unsweetened fruits in their own juices.) Cook up a few different frozen or fresh vegetables and have them waiting for you in plastic containers. Make a huge lettuce, tomato, cucumber, red pepper, and onion salad with vinegar and spices. Let it stand overnight. It will taste delicious. Broil turkey or chicken breasts and wrap them in foil and refrigerate. Make a large tuna salad with chopped cucumber, onion, celery, and lemon juice or a tablespoon of low-fat mayonnaise. When you come home from work starving, you can dig in without waiting two minutes—and no harm will be done to your diet.

If you have a little more restraint when you come home starving, it only takes 15 minutes to broil flounder or sole while simultaneously cooking frozen vegetables and pasta. (You can have four ounces of spaghetti sauce on your pasta, as long as it has less than 75 calories for four ounces—check the label.)

SAMPLE WEIGHT-LOSS DIET

BREAKFAST

One poached egg or two-thirds cup plain oatmeal

One slice whole-wheat toast or one-half bran muffin

No-calorie beverage

Six ounces glass of juice or one fruit

Coffee or tea (decaffeinated—optional)

LUNCH

Chef salad without beef, ham, or cheese *or*

White-meat turkey sandwich with lettuce and tomato on whole-wheat bread *or*

Water-packed tuna sandwich (mix tuna with various chopped vegetables, spices, and lemon or vinegar)

Tossed salad, vinegar and spices dressing

One cup any allowed fresh or frozen vegetable

DINNER

Six to eight ounces of any low-fat fish listed above, or white-meat turkey or chicken

One potato with low-fat plain yogurt as a sour cream substitute *or*

Four ounces protein or whole-wheat spaghetti with four ounces tomato sauce

One or two cups any vegetables

Tossed salad

No-calorie beverage

SNACKS

There's no reason to ever deny yourself food when you're feeling hungry. In fact, I want you to make it your business to eat at least two snacks (the right ones, of course) in addition to your three meals. Every time you eat, your metabolism goes "on" and begins burning calories. If you eat low-calorie snacks, your body usually burns more calories than the snack itself provides, and you end up losing more weight. When you don't eat for long periods of time, your metabolism slows down and you burn very few calories. The end result is you go hungry and you lose less weight than you would have had you snacked. Try not to go more than four hours without eating. (I eat more often than that.)

You can have a cup of cooked or raw vegetables any time of the day or night. I like to cut up two cucumbers and douse them with vinegar, or have a cup or two of steamed vegetables. Red peppers are delicious, and I'll eat two or three at a time. Except for potatoes and corn, don't worry about the calories of vegetables when you have them as snacks. On this diet, they are virtually "free."

You can have two to three fruits a day if you need a quick energy spurt. Think of each fruit as about 100 calories.

No-calorie beverages are always allowed, and if you really crave something sweet, you can satisfy your sweet tooth and have a slice of whole-wheat toast with one or two teaspoons of regular sugary jelly or jam (16 calories a teaspoon). But be careful. You'll probably want more in 20 minutes. When that happens control yourself. Say to yourself, "I realize this urge is a result of the sugar." Then eat a piece of fruit instead.

HOW TO KEEP YOUR DIET WHILE EATING ON THE RUN: THE FAT-BURNING, EAT-ANYWHERE DIET

You can eat on the run and still keep your diet. Certain allowances can be made when you are not able to obtain "ideal" foods. As long as you don't eat the * foods more than twice a week, you will not damage your nutritious weight-loss plan. I eat this way at least twice a week and, frankly, I'm glad. Eating "straight" all the time is sooo boring.

BREAKFAST

Have one-half large bran *or* corn muffin* *or* one-half bagel* *or* one-half English muffin* with 1 teaspoon of butter, jelly, or cream cheese. (Yes, that's right. The whole deal amounts to no more than 200 calories, no matter which you choose.) Or you can grab one or two slices of whole-wheat bread and an orange and eat them on the way to work, or have them with coffee at work, if you can't stop to buy or order the above.

Don't skip breakfast. It will *not* help you to lose weight.

LUNCH

Have eight ounces of low-fat cottage cheese, *or* eight ounces of low-fat yogurt (any flavor, but plain is lowest in calories), *or* one slice of pizza* with fat blotted off, *or* one large soft pretzel,* *or* a bowl of soup with crackers. Drink a low-calorie beverage, and finish your meal with a piece of fruit or a half-ounce box of raisins.*

DINNER

Have a white-meat turkey or chicken hero* with lettuce, tomatoes, and mustard, *or* a white-meat turkey sandwich on whole-wheat toast, *or* a serving of linguini* with red clam sauce and tossed salad, *or* eight ounces low-fat cottage cheese and a fruit.

SNACKS

Pick one choice from among fruit, yogurt, and hard-boiled egg. You can have raw vegetables anytime.

WHEN YOU'RE DESPERATE

You can have a hot dog. The calories won't kill you (about 400 calories for everything) but the food content may if you do it more than once every other month. You can have a fast-food hamburger (no cheese) if you blot it thoroughly with a napkin first. Don't do this more than once every two weeks while you're dieting, however. Do it only in an "extreme emergency."

KEEPING
YOUR DIET AT A PARTY

You don't have to dread going to parties. You can eat and drink along with everyone else, only you'll have to be selective. If you choose to drink alcoholic beverages, stick to champagne or white wine. If you prefer the "hard stuff," have one or two glasses of vodka with club soda. No matter what you choose to drink, have it with water, club soda, grapefruit juice, or orange juice—in that order of preference. Of course, if you're trying to lose weight, it's better to stay away from alcoholic beverages altogether. I do, except for a glass or two of champagne, which I'll have if I'm in the mood, even when I'm on the strictest diet.

You can nibble on the raw vegetables, but forgo the dip, which is solid fat (sour cream is the base). If chicken or turkey is served, choose the white meat and remove any skin. Avoid beef, cheese, and ham. You can have plain salad, pickles (high in sodium but low in calories) and peppers, but avoid the olives (high in oil). You can indeed eat the bread, even white if whole-wheat is not available. A little compromise will not ruin your diet. Generally try to follow the eating guidelines presented in this chapter. You'll be surprised to see how easy it is. No one will even notice that you're dieting, unless you make an announcement.

Eating and Enjoying Your "Forbidden Foods"

Once you have reached your goal weight, you can eat virtually anything you want (given, of course, any restrictions from your doctor regarding your particular health problems), but you'll have to pace yourself. Eat any of the foods listed above in the carbohydrate and protein categories—including the high-calorie items. However, if you like red meat, limit your intake to once a week. Do observe a rough calorie limit—your daily calorie consumption can now rise to about 2,000—but don't count calories. Just be aware. If you drink alcoholic beverages, you can now have a drink or two once or twice a week, but don't mix alcohol with anything other than club soda, except on your free eating day, if you so choose. It's generally best to stick to white wine or champagne.

Your Free Eating Day

Choose one day a week and eat anything you please. You can have a banana split, a greasy hamburger, doughnuts, chocolate candy or ice-cream—any and all of them. As long as you return to good eating habits the other six days of the week, you won't gain weight.

PLANNING YOUR FREE EATING DAY

It's a good idea to think ahead. If there's a special occasion coming up, such as a holiday or a special dinner engagement, save your free day for that event. This way you won't have to worry about working around the food served. If you eat wildly for more than one day, then watch your diet for a week for each "naughty" day. In other words, don't take advantage of another free eating day until you have made up the number of weeks for each day you indulged.

Now turn to Chapter 12 to find out how to keep your diet when you're dining out and/or are away from home.

NOTES

[1] Patricia Hausman, *The Calcium Bible,* New York: Rawson Associates, 1985, pg. 123.

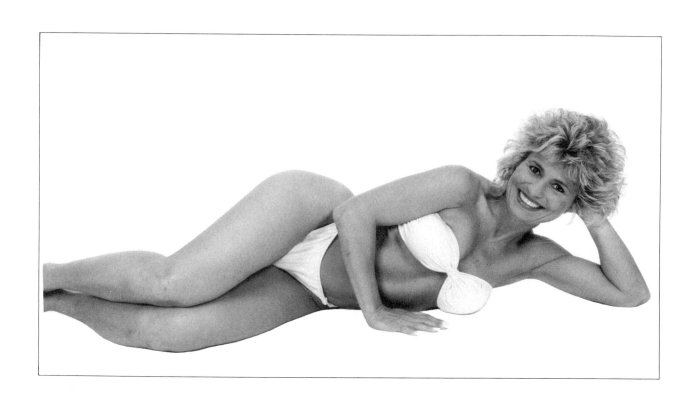

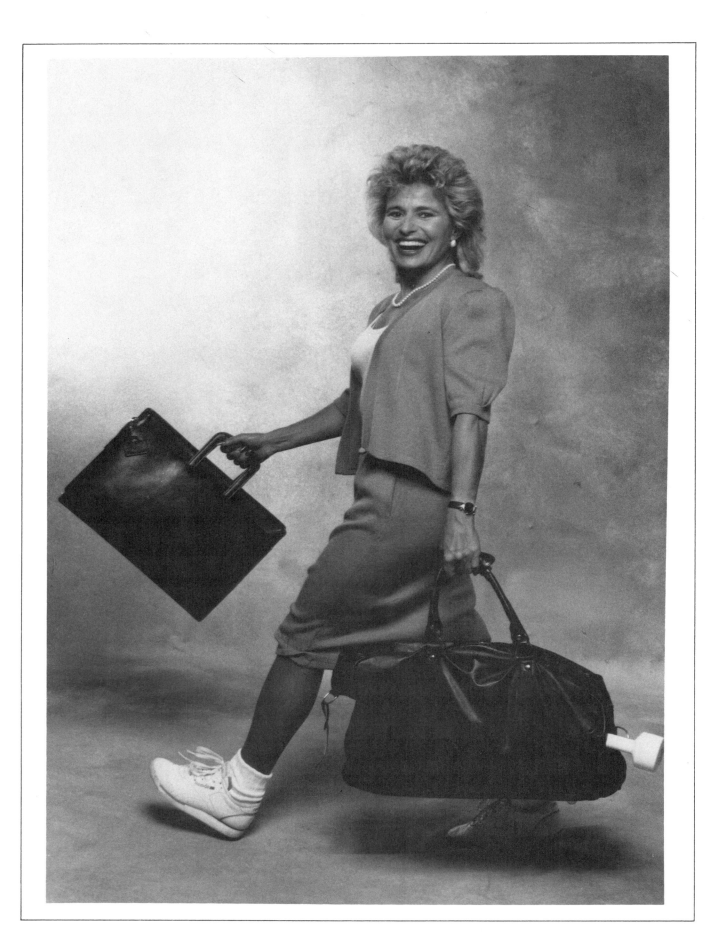

12

ON THE ROAD AGAIN

The problem with most fitness programs is that you can't take them with you! This program is different. You can both work out and keep your diet, whether you're on a business trip or a vacation—anywhere in the world. All you need are your three-pound dumbbells and your fitness mentality.

YOUR ON-THE-ROAD MENTALITY

When a person is about to go out of town, it's not unusual for him or her to think, I'm going away. Oh well, there goes all my hard work. I hate to think of what I'll have to do to get back in shape when I return home.

People think this way because they're conditioned to believe that when they leave their home base, they must also leave self-direction behind. They envision difficulties in finding time and space to work out, and anticipate problems obtaining appropriate foods, so they adopt a "victim" attitude and assume that they must allow themselves to be controlled by the environment instead of realizing that *they can be in control* of it.

Imagine what a relief it would be to you if you found out that you could not only maintain your fitness program on the road, but that it's even easier to diet and work out when you're away than when you are at home.

KEEPING YOUR DIET AND WORKING OUT IS EASIER WHEN YOU'RE AWAY FROM HOME

THE REFRIGERATOR IS NOT AVAILABLE

Whenever you travel, you can actually lose weight. You don't have to try to do this—all you have to do is take advantage of the natural flow of things. For example, when you're on the road, you don't have access to your refrigerator. In order to get something to eat, you have to make a special effort—you must either order room service or go into a restaurant and order food. When I'm on the road, for example, if I have an urge for an after-dinner snack even though I'm not really hungry, it's much easier for me not to call room service than it is for me not to go to a refrigerator. When I don't indulge before bedtime, I wake up in the morning feeling refreshed and energetic, because I have an empty stomach. After doing this for a few nights, I lose weight. It's my hotel travel experiences that make me realize how easy it would be to keep my weight down if I simply refused to eat any food after dinner at home. But that's not easy for me, so I just take advantage of my travel time.

WHEN YOU'RE DINING IN PUBLIC, YOU MAINTAIN MORE CONTROL

When you're in public, you tend to eat less than when you're in the privacy of your own home. For example, at a self-service banquet, even if you fill your plate to overflowing, unless you go back for second and third helpings, you'll probably eat a lot less than you eat at a home dinner. If you're like most people, when you're at home and no one is around to see you, you "pig out" on second and third helpings. Most people eat with two forks when no one is around, and some don't even bother with forks. They stand in front of the opened refrigerator and eat with their hands until their heart's content.

If you want to make sure you don't go back for second and third helpings, try to conduct business at the banquet dinner, or at least sit with someone with whom you can carry on a stimulating conversation. When dessert is served, have coffee and fruit or a piece of bread or just coffee. No one really cares whether or not you indulge. If they comment on the fact that you're not eating dessert, it's because they wish they had your discipline.

WORKING OUT IS EASIER ON THE ROAD

When you're in a strange situation, you have to set new routines for everything from basic hygiene to getting dressed in the morning. Since everything is different anyway, it's easy to incorporate your workout into your day. Later, I'll suggest specific ways to do it.

CARRYING THE DUMBBELLS

Put the dumbbells at the bottom of your suitcase, one on each side for balance. If you're traveling very light, you can place them in your attaché or briefcase. The six pounds of added weight will help you burn some additional fat as you carry your bag from place to place.

I don't recommend leaving the dumbbells at home and buying a pair when you get to your destination. Carrying the dumbbells is important to your mental attitude. It's a symbol of your fitness mentality. If you think six pounds is too much excess baggage, realize that at one point of your life you were probably carrying around at least six pounds of extra fat. In fact, maybe you are right now, and you manage to do it every day—all day. You can handle the dumbbells with no real problem.

WHAT TO EAT ON THE PLANE

There's no reason to submit yourself humbly to whatever is served to you on the plane. If you call 24 hours in advance, most airlines will provide you with a variety of special menus. Several major airlines offer a choice of seafood, vegetarian, low-calorie, low-sodium, and low-fat entrées.

The best choices are the low-sodium, low-fat, or low-calorie meals. A sample low-sodium breakfast consists of orange juice, an omelet (blot the omelet with a napkin to remove any oil), a tomato wedge, and wafers. One low-fat lunch is made up of lean meat, seafood, or poultry without the skin, vegetables cooked without oil or butter, and a fruit. A sample low-calorie dinner is chicken breast (no skin), broccoli and carrots (prepared with little or no butter or oil), lettuce, tomato and cucumber salad, and fresh melon in season.

If you choose seafood or vegetarian entrées, beware of any visible oil or fat. For example, one seafood platter that can sometimes be ordered for lunch or dinner is tomato stuffed with crabmeat, shrimp, artichoke hearts, cocktail sauce on the side, and a salad with dressing on the side. You can blot the shrimp if it's been fried and forgo the salad dressing, but you can have the cocktail sauce. It isn't very fattening. An example of a vegetarian meal is grilled tomato, leaf spinach, melba-peach half, whole-wheat bread, and yogurt. You can blot off any excess oil from the tomato and check the spinach for excess butter. The peach-melba half is okay, even if it does have a little sugar on it, and yogurt is always acceptable.

When you call the airline to order your special meal, ask them to give you a list of their low-calorie, low-fat offerings, and then ask them to specify what foods will be served in a given meal. They usually have such information available in their computers.

What if you forget to call ahead? You can work around the food that is served. Most airlines give choices of beef, chicken, or fish. Choose the chicken or fish. Remove the skin from the chicken and blot off excess fat from the chicken or fish with a napkin. (The fish or chicken may have been broiled with butter or oil.) If the vegetables appear to be buttery, spoon them into a napkin to remove the excess fat, then clean the excess butter from the vegetable portion of your plate with a napkin and return the vegetables to the plate. You can smile broadly with a twinkle in your eye if your seat companion gives you a strange look, and then continue to do what you're doing. Unless he or she is paying your rent, you owe no explanation. You can eat your salad with no problem. The dressing is always on the side. Any low- or no-calorie drink is fair game.

Unless you're celebrating something very special and want to mark the occasion with a glass of champagne, avoid alcoholic beverages on planes. Their effect seems to double on a plane, and if you indulge even in one or two drinks, you can count on a hangover descending upon your head with the landing of the plane, and that's no fun.

WORKING OUT ON THE PLANE

You don't have to work out on the plane. You can stretch out or walk around a few times if you're so inclined. However, if the flight is longer than three hours, you can perform one exercise for each body part, doing them without the dumbbells. The movements performed with isometric pressure and dynamic tension alone will provide enough stimulation to help relieve built-up tension. After such a workout, you'll be able to sit and read for another hour or so. If the flight is long, you may want to do a 12-minute routine every few hours.

THE 12-MINUTE WORKOUT ON THE ROAD

The best time to work out when you're on the road is first thing in the morning, before you have time to negotiate the issue—even before you brush your teeth or shower.

If you know you have the self-discipline, however, and you anticipate an afternoon break when working out will be convenient for you and will help to relieve midday tension, you can postpone it until that time.

Some people like to work out in the evening, about an hour before bedtime. I hate to leave anything so important for the end of the day, because if something comes up, there's no way to make it up later. But you know your routines, so working out late at night may work well for you.

The beauty of this workout is its flexibility. Even if your wake-up call never comes and you're forced to skip your usual morning workout, you can always find 12 minutes in the day to fit it in. There's practically no reason ever to skip a workout. (See page 38, however, for what to do if you do skip a workout.)

AEROBICS

You can do two of your three 20-minute aerobic sessions on the weekends, if your on-the-road schedule is conducive to more free time then, and fit the other one in on a Wednesday or Thursday morning or evening, right after you perform your 12-minute workout. You won't be too tired to run, jump rope, swim, or walk, because aerobics have an energizing effect.

I like either to jump rope in my room in the morning while watching the news on television or listening to soft music on the radio, or to go outside and run 10 minutes in one direction, then turn around and head back to the hotel. If you choose to walk instead of run, walk 20 minutes in each direction.

If the hotel offers aerobics classes, you can get your aerobics done while meeting interesting people at the same time—assuming, of course, the class happens to fit your schedule. If the hotel has a pool, you can swim for 20 minutes. Forty minutes of tennis will also cover a 20-minute aerobics session.

EXERCISE SPURTS ON THE ROAD

It's important to remember to fit in at least one or two 12-minute exercise spurts during the day when you're away from home, whether you're on vacation or on a business trip. (You need less than the usual three, because most people are more active when they're away from home.) If you're on a business trip, you can make it a point to take a short walk, six minutes in each direction, before and/or after lunch or during a meeting break.

Another way to get in an exercise spurt on the road is to return to your room and do 12 minutes of jumping jacks or calisthenic-type exercises.

SKIPPING A WORKOUT: WHAT SHOULD I SKIP?

If your schedule is very tight and you can only afford to do the bare minimum of exercise while you're on the road, your priority should be lined up in this order:

1. A 12-minute total-body workout

2. Two additional exercise spurts of 12 minutes during day

3. Three 20-minute aerobic sessions

VACATIONS FROM THIS WORKOUT

"Do I ever get a vacation from this workout?" you may wonder. Yes. You can take a few weeks off a year with no consequence whatsoever. It's better to take time off one week at a time, if possible. In any case, after laying off for a week or two, you will miss the workout and will be eager to start up again.

EATING OUT ON THE ROAD

If you're staying in a hotel, you'll have to deal with four food offerings: breakfast, lunch, and dinner restaurant menus, and room service menus. I've traveled back and forth across the United States for weeks at a time, staying in a wide range of hotels, and I've discovered that there's always something palatable to order from the menu—if you know what you are doing. The purpose of this section is to provide a guideline as to what is and what is not acceptable fare when seeking to keep your diet on the road. I've selected as my sample hotels: Holiday Inn, Omni International, Westin, and Marriott, and I've chosen limited, moderate, and unlimited menus so that you can anticipate a variety of problems such as typically come up when ordering food in hotels.

When a hotel menu is limited, your problem is finding something to eat without breaking your diet. When the menu is replete with choices, your problem is the same: finding something to eat without breaking your diet. The following paragraphs will tell you how you can find *something* to eat, even in the most limiting circumstances, and what to avoid when the menu offering is endless.

A given hotel menu may vary from one season to another, so keep in mind that the menus discussed here may not be exactly the same if you should visit the named hotels at some time in the future. The purpose of this section is not to limit your thinking to one hotel or one menu, but to show you that every hotel and every menu can be worked around so that you can maintain good eating habits when you're away from home. I selected these particular hotels because I have spent time in each of them, and because they were particularly cooperative in supplying me with menus. After reading this section, you should understand the basic principles of food selection when dining out, so that you will be able to stay in any hotel or motel, anywhere in the world, no matter how unlimited or limited the menu, and still keep your diet.

BREAKFAST: HOLIDAY INN—RUNNEMEDE, NEW JERSEY (Limited Menu)

FRUITS AND JUICES:

Assorted juices*

Half a fresh grapefruit*

Melon in season*

EGGS AND OMELETS:

One or two eggs any style*

Breakfast steak with eggs any style
(served with toast and home fries)

Three-egg omelet: plain, ham, cheese, western
(all omelets served with toast and home fries)

CONTINENTAL BREAKFAST:

Choice of juice*

Danish or English muffin and beverage**

Bagel and cream cheese**

Juice and beverage*

PANCAKES AND
FRENCH TOAST:

Short or full stack of pancakes

French toast

Waffles

SIDE ORDERS:

English muffin, assorted Danish, or bagel**

Bacon, breakfast ham, sausage

Toast*

Breakfast steak is beef, and too high in fat. Home fries are cooked with oil, and omelets are cooked with cheese, butter, and other fattening ingredients. Avoid them. Danishes, pancakes, French toast, and waffles contain processed carbohydrates and high fat. Bacon, sausages, and ham are high in fat. Never eat them when you're dieting.

If you choose a food marked with **, there are limitations. You may have a half a bagel and one tablespoon of cream cheese, or you may have half an English muffin with a tablespoon of jelly or a pat of butter.

If you order eggs, make sure they're either poached, hard-boiled, or soft-boiled. All other eggs will be cooked in butter. *All foods marked * are perfect if you're trying to lose weight.*

LUNCH: THE WESTIN BONAVENTURE, LOS ANGELES, CALIFORNIA (Unlimited Menu)

FRESH STARTERS:

Breaded fried chicken strips and drumettes

Deep-fried mozzarella, shrimp, zucchini sticks, and onion rings

Half papaya with fresh fruit*

Shrimp cocktail*

Smoked fish plate

Whole fresh artichoke with julienne of vegetables, basil vinaigrette**

Calzone with prosciutto and Sonoma goat cheese

Whenever you see the word *fried* on any menu, move on to the next item. Smoked anything is high in both calories and sodium. Calzone with prosciutto and goat cheese is unacceptable, as are most cheese dishes because of their high fat content. You may choose from the papaya and fresh fruit, the fruit cocktail, or the artichoke dish (without the vinaigrette dressing—it contains oil).

SOUPS:

Fish soup*

Soup of the day

Baked onion soup

Onion soup is always high in fat, but the fish soup is okay, except for the fact that all soups are very high in sodium, and it's uncomfortable to retain water when you're on the road.

FRESH SALADS

Salad bar**

Seafood salad**

Tostada salad

Pasta salad with fresh vegetables, ham, and turkey

Chicken and tuna salad served with avocados and tomatoes

Sliced fruit and berries, choice of sherbet, yogurt, or low-fat yogurt*

The tostada salad is high in calories—too much oil in the tostadas. Avoid pasta salad; it's usually tossed in an oily dressing. Chicken and tuna salad are made with mayonnaise, which is pure fat.

The salad bar is a good idea, but use only plain vinegar or lemon as dressing. Leave the croutons and the olives, and avoid all cheeses (except cottage cheese, but limit yourself to two-thirds cup). Pickles are okay, except they are high in sodium. Most other items in a salad bar are acceptable, but be aware of the general rules of good eating as discussed in Chapter 11.

If you choose the seafood salad, be aware that it usually comes with an oily dressing, so order the dressing on the side and ask for plain vinegar.

(You may want to use one tablespoon of the dressing and add vinegar to the salad.) If you order the sliced fruit dish, be sure to get the low-fat yogurt with it.

FRESH PASTAS

Tomato fettuccine with poached salmon and smoked salmon dill in cream sauce

Spinach fettuccine with szechuan style duck strips

Vegetable lasagna*

Linguini with shrimp, mushroom, or cream sauce*

As soon as you see the words *cream* or *duck*, move to the next item. They are both almost pure fat. The vegetable lasagna is an excellent choice, or you can order the linguini with shrimp or mushroom sauce. Ask the waiter if they have red clam sauce with the linguine. It's delicious and low in calories.

FRESH CATCH:

Cajun style red snapper**

Grilled swordfish steak, ginger lime sauce**

Sautéed salmon, dill butter

Scallops with fennel sauce*

Steamed trout, julienne of vegetables

Tempura fried shrimp with zucchini, soy sauce

Red snapper is high in calories, and the sauce will add more calories. But it's still not a cream sauce, and it is fish, so you can order it if you're close to your weight goal. If you choose the grilled swordfish, order it grilled with lemon instead of ginger lime sauce (too high in fat). You can do the same for the salmon. However, both swordfish and salmon are rather high-fat fishes, so are best avoided unless you're close to your weight goal. The fried shrimp is out of the question for obvious reasons, so the steamed trout dish is your best bet.

FRESH GROUND BURGERS:

I won't even list the choices. Beef is too high in calories for a weight-loss diet.

FRESH SANDWICHES:

The Westin Club*

Vegetarian pita, filled with fresh mushrooms, tomatoes, cucumbers, alfalfa sprouts, cream cheese and walnuts*

Turkey, ham, and cheese croissant

Philadelphia cheese steak (thinly sliced New York sirloin topped with melted cheddar cheese, served with French roll)

You know why ham, cheese, and steak are not acceptable choices. You can choose either the Westin club (if you order it with white-meat turkey or chicken on whole-wheat with lettuce and tomatoes, and no mayonnaise), or the vegetarian pita (remove the cream cheese and walnuts of course—fat and oil)

FRESH ENTRÉES:

Stir-fry chicken, snow peas with mushrooms, fried rice

Stir-fry beef and chicken combination, fried rice

Gourmet pizza with your choice of shrimp or topping of the day**

Chicken with beef fajitas, served with tortillas

Sautéed chicken breast with mushrooms and blue corn pancakes

Don't be fooled by the word *stir* when it appears next to *fry*. *Fry*ing still requires oil, which is fat, and fried rice is out of the question, as is beef. Tortillas are high in fat. Beware of "sautéed" dishes—they often contain lots of fat; so ask the waiter to tell you exactly what the chicken is sautéed in. Don't eat the pancakes. The only possibility here, believe it or not, is the pizza, if they have vegetarian pizza and you blot it carefully with some napkins. Tell them to go very light on the cheese, or to eliminate it altogether if possible.

FROM THE GRILL:

All steaks are out of the question. No need to discuss.

FRESH HEALTH PLATTERS:

Grilled range-fed half chicken with lemon sauce*

Baked halibut with hazelnut butter**

Heart of artichoke salad with slices of chicken breast, basil vinaigrette*

Crabmeat sandwich on white or whole-wheat bread*

Beware of the words *health* or *diet* on any menu. The foods are often quite fattening. There are things on the above list, however, that you can eat if you make a few changes. You could ask for the crabmeat sandwich on whole-wheat bread—without the mayonnaise it's usually mixed with—or you can order the chicken (remove the skin, and eliminate the sauce). You can have the halibut if you eliminate the hazelnut butter. The heart of artichoke salad is fine, if you exchange the vinaigrette for plain vinegar.

FRESH SWEETS AND TREATS:

This category is for later, when you indulge in your free eating day.

FRESH CHEESES:

No cheese until you reach your weight goal.

DINNER: MARRIOTT–ASHLEY'S
(Moderate Offering)

APPETIZERS:

Shrimp cocktail (large shrimp with a chilled lemon dill mayonnaise and zesty cocktail sauce)*

Gravlax (rosettes of fresh cured salmon served with capers, chopped egg, onion, and croutons)

Baked oysters Thermidor (plump oysters, with sliced mushrooms and lobster topped with a sherry cream sauce)

Smoked duck breast (served with a cranberry chutney)

Crab Hoezell (backfin crabmeat with tarragon vinegar and olive oil)

Wild game sausage (served with a gingered piquante sauce)

Shrimp Beradi (butterflied shrimp with provolone cheese wrapped in cured ham, and baked with Dijon butter)

Pasta and shiitake mushrooms (tomato pasta with shiitake mushrooms in a seasoned cream sauce)

Unless you want a shrimp cocktail without the mayonnaise, I'd skip the appetizers altogether and simply have a salad. Most of the other appetizers are prepared in fattening sauces, and cannot be ordered with sauce on the side without destroying the essence of the dish. The duck, sausage, and ham, as you know, are too high in fat.

SALADS:

Warm spinach salad (fresh spinach tossed with bay shrimp, chopped egg, and bacon, served with warm honey vinaigrette dressing)*

Tomato and goat cheese (thick slices of tomato and sweet onion topped with goat cheese and accompanied with capers and a vinaigrette dressing)

The spinach salad is perfect, if you can resist eating the bacon, and you don't have the dressing. Use vinegar or lemon juice and spices. The goat cheese dish is out for obvious reasons.

ENTRÉES FROM THE GRILL:

All entrées include Ashley's salad,* fresh vegetables,* and choice of potato or rice*.

Grilled salmon (fresh grilled and served with a champagne and whole-grain mustard sauce)**

Mixed grill (combination of broiled chicken breast, duck breast, and shrimp served with a honey amaretto sauce, sherry sauce, and juniper sauce)

Sirloin strip steak

Filet mignon

Grilled swordfish (served with a tomato herb coulis)**

Mixed grill of seafood (a combination of our freshest seafood)*

Order your salad with plain vinegar on the side, and your vegetables cooked with no butter. Either a plain baked potato or plain rice are acceptable. You can ask for plain yogurt to be used in place of sour cream on the potato.

The mixed grill is not acceptable because of the duck and the honey sauce, and the sirloin steak and filet mignon are beef and are too high in fat. Salmon and swordfish are high-fat fishes but are still much lower in fat than beef. In this case, you can even have them with their low-fat sauces if you're close to your weight goal.

SPECIALTIES:

Lobster Chemise (lobster wrapped in flavored spinach and puff pastry, served on a bed of saffron cream sauce)

Rack of Lamb (baked in a crust and served with port wine sauce)

Cajun barbecued shrimp (large shrimp sautéed in New Orleans spices and served with a French baguette for dipping)

Crab cakes Chesapeake (deep-fried lump crabmeat served on a bed of creamy Old Bay sauce)

Dover sole (sautéed with capers, lemon zest, fresh parsley, and butter)*

Veal medallions (sautéed with wild mushrooms and served with herbed pasta)

Chicken tarragon (marinated breast of chicken grilled and glazed with a light white-wine sauce with shallots and tarragon)*

Veal milan (medallions sautéed and topped with ricotta cheese, spinach, sun-dried tomatoes, and fresh sauce)

The Cajun shrimp is out because you won't be able to dip the baguette into the fattening sauce and that's no fun. Veal is beef, and it's too high in fat. That leaves you with two choices: Dover sole or chicken tarragon. Ask the waiter if the lemon "zest" contains butter or oil. If it does, ask to have the fish broiled in lemon only. You can enjoy the chicken tarragon as it is.

ROOM SERVICE: THE OMNI INTERNATIONAL HOTEL, DETROIT, MICHIGAN (Moderate Choices)

Since room service in most hotels offers similar breakfast, lunch, and dinner menus, as do their restaurants, and we've already discussed those, I'll limit my discussion to all-day and late-night offerings.

ALL-DAY PIZZAS:

Farmers cheese, prosciutto, tomato, artichokes, basil, and garlic

Shrimp and pesto pizza with fresh tomato, shrimp, pesto, parmesan cheese, and artichokes**

Three-cheese pizza with jack, chevre, and colby cheese with tomatoes, oregano, garlic, and olive oil

The farmers cheese and three-cheese pizzas are too "cheesey" for diet purposes, but you could order the shrimp and pesto pizza if you're willing to thoroughly blot the pizza with a napkin to remove excess oil. You can also ask the cook to go very light on the parmesan cheese and heavy on the tomatoes.

DESSERTS:

Grand Marnier custard

Fresh fruit flan

Fresh seasonal berries*

Selection of Haagen Dazs ice-creams and sorbets

Chocolate genache torte

Chef's mousse

Your only choice here is the berries. You can sprinkle NutraSweet over them for a delicious treat.

ALL-DAY SNACKS:

Mixed nuts, bowl

Potato chips, bowl

Pretzels, bowl**

Doritos chips, bowl

Onion dip

Fried mozzarella cheese with picante sauce

Buffalo chicken wings with blue cheese dip

Deep-fried onion rings

French fries

Cottage cheese*

Domestic fruits and cheese*

Nuts, potato chips, and Doritos are high in fat. Onion dip is made with sour cream. Mozzarella cheese is high in fat, and buffalo chicken wings, onion rings, and french fries are all high in fat. You can have the pretzels. They're only about 100 calories an ounce, but they're a bit high in sodium. Cottage cheese or domestic fruit is your best bet, but of course, order the fruit *without* the cheese.

Although it isn't listed, most hotels' room services will make you a plain or chef's salad. (Order the chef's salad without the ham and beef.)

LATE-NIGHT APPETIZERS:

Smoked white fish chowder**

333 East onion soup

Steamed gulf shrimp with cocktail sauce*

Onion soup is too high in fat, but you can have the fish chowder if you don't mind retaining a little water. The best choice is the steamed gulf shrimp, and you can even have the cocktail sauce with no guilt.

SALADS:

333 East mixed green salad with choice of basil, honey poppy seed, blue cheese, mustard basil, or Marie Rose dressing*

Cobb Salad (Boston and romaine lettuce, spinach, country ham, turkey, Swiss and cheddar cheese, tossed with Brown Derby dressing)*

The mixed green salad is ideal, but order two dressings on the side to choose from, plus plain vinegar. Then use only one tablespoon of the dressing and add two or three tablespoons of vinegar so that the dressing can cover your entire salad. *Delicious and no guilt* because no matter how fattening the dressing is, if you only use one tablespoon, it can't be more than 100 calories. The vinegar is virtually calorie-free.

The Cobb salad is fine if you get the dressing on the side and eliminate the ham and cheeses. (They will give you extra turkey instead.) Use one tablespoon of dressing and add vinegar as described above.

THE CARNEGIE DELI:

Lean pastrami with Swiss cheese, served on rye bread with mustard

Tuna salad with sliced egg on an onion roll

Turkey breast on whole-wheat*

Ham and Swiss cheese on rye bread

There's no such thing as "lean" pastrami. Don't believe it for a second. It's beef and it's fatty. Tuna salad is made with mayonnaise, and ham and cheese are too high in fat. An excellent choice is the turkey breast on whole-wheat. This is perfect for even the most strict diets. You can ask for mustard and lettuce and tomatoes on the side, and then make the sandwich to suit your taste. Mustard is slightly high in sodium, but you can indulge without guilt if you've generally been keeping your sodium low.

PICKING AND CHOOSING

If your goal is to lose weight as fast as possible, choose only the * foods. If you're almost at goal or on maintenance, you may also cautiously choose from the ** category. If you're indulging in your free eating day, you can of course eat anything you wish.

No matter how limited a hotel menu is, there's always something you can eat. Here are some foods that you can get in virtually any hotel, whether or not they are on the menu.

Eggs—poached or hard- or soft-boiled

A lettuce and tomato salad

A chef's salad (with white-meat turkey and hard-boiled eggs)

Whole-wheat toast

Broiled chicken, flounder, or sole

Baked potato

Plain white rice

Shrimp cocktail

Fruit

Various vegetables—raw and cooked

ON THE RUN ON THE ROAD

If you're on the road, on the run, in the middle of nowhere, and you see a small deli or grocery store, you can get any of the following to tide you over: white-meat turkey or chicken breast sandwich on whole-wheat bread; tomato-and-lettuce sandwich with one tablespoon of mayonnaise (the calories in the sandwich are so low, you can afford to splurge on the mayonnaise); an eight-ounce container of low-fat yogurt or cottage cheese; fruit; raw carrots; celery; red or green peppers; cucumbers; a white-meat turkey hero**; a bag of pretzels (low-sodium if possible).

FOREIGN COUNTRIES

No matter where you are in the world, they're likely to have fruits, vegetables, poultry, and fish. Order foods within the limitations of the situation, and stick to the guidelines above and those discussed in Chapter 11. I've traveled all over Europe, Africa, and South America, and I've been able to maintain good eating habits.

Of course, if you're on vacation, you may want to abandon your regimen for a week or two, but frankly, I wouldn't throw all caution to the wind for more than a week at a time. It's not necessary and, after a week, it's not even fun. Your body will be the first to let you know that it craves nutritious foods, because you'll begin to feel lethargic and even irritable. You'll have a much better time if you pay attention to those signals and begin eating right again.

A FINAL WORD

I know the power of this program to solve your fitness problems, but it always delights me to hear from you. Please write and let me know how you're doing. Address your letter to:

> Joyce L. Vedral
> P.O. Box A433
> Wantagh, NY 11793-0433

The same address can be used to order a pair of my cast-iron three pound dumbbells. Enclose a check or money order for $12.00. You will pay U.P.S. charges upon receipt.

You may order a set of three pound water-weights for weight-free travel by calling CAEF Inc. 1-800-635-8132.

BIBLIOGRAPHY

EXERCISE BOOKS FOR ADDITIONAL TRAINING

McLish, Rachel, and Joyce L. Vedral, Ph.D. *Perfect Parts.* New York: Warner Books, 1987.

Portugues, Gladys, and Joyce L. Vedral, Ph.D. *Hard Bodies.* New York: Dell Publishing, 1986.

Portugues, Gladys, and Joyce L. Vedral, Ph.D. *Hard Bodies Express Workout.* New York: Dell Publishing, 1988.

Vedral, Joyce, Ph.D. *Now or Never.* New York: Warner Books, 1986.

NUTRITION BOOKS FOR ADDITIONAL INFORMATION

Hausman, Patricia, M.S. *The Calcium Bible.* New York: Rawson Associates, 1985.

Kirshbaum, John (ed.). *The Nutrition Almanac.* New York: McGraw-Hill, 1984.

LeGette, Bernard. *LeGette's Calorie Encyclopedia.* New York: Warner Books, 1983.

Liebman, Bonnie F., Michael Jacobson, M.D., and Greg Moyer. *Salt: The Brand Name Guide to Sodium Content.* New York: Warner Books, 1983.

Mindell, Earl. *Earl Mindell's New and Revised Vitamin Bible.* New York: Warner Books, 1985.

Netzer, Corinne T. *The Dieter's Calorie Counter.* New York: Dell Publishing, 1983.

Reynolds, Bill, and Joyce Vedral, Ph.D. *Supercut: Nutrition for the Ultimate Physique.* Chicago: Contemporary Books, 1985.

Tatum, Dr. Kermit R. *Shake the Salt Habit*. New York: Ballantine Books, 1981.

Vaughan, Dr. William. *Low Sugar Secrets for Your Diet*. New York: Warner Books, 1985.

MEDICAL BOOKS FOR ADDITIONAL INFORMATION

Borysenko, Joan, Ph.D. *Minding the Body, Mending the Mind*. Reading, Massachusetts: Addison-Wesley Publishing, 1987.

Ornstein, Robert, Ph.D. and David Sobel, M.D. *The Healing Brain*. New York: Simon & Schuster, 1987.

Siegel, Bernie W., M.D. *Love, Medicine and Miracles*. New York: Harper & Row, 1986.

ABOUT THE AUTHOR

Joyce Vedral has written and co-authored several books on fitness: *Now or Never, Perfect Parts* (with Rachel McLish), *Hard Bodies* (with Gladys Portugues), *The Hard Bodies Express Workout* (with Gladys Portugues), and *Supercut: Nutrition for the Ultimate Physique* (with Bill Reynolds). She gives lectures and holds fitness seminars throughout the United States.

In addition to her fitness pursuits, Joyce teaches English to young adults, and is the author of several best-selling self-help books for that age group: *I Dare You, My Parents Are Driving Me Crazy, I Can't Take It Any More,* and *The Opposite Sex Is Driving Me Crazy.*

A Ph.D. in English Literature (New York University), Joyce has been actively involved in both the martial arts and bodybuilding for a number of years. She holds a brown belt in Kodokon Judo, a green belt in Jui-Jitsu, and a brown belt in Go-Ju Karate. She has worked with champion bodybuilders for the past 10 years, interviewing them for *Muscle and Fitness* and *Shape* magazines, and has competed in and won prizes in various physique championships, including "Most Muscular" and "Best Abdominals." She has recently been featured in *Female Bodybuilding* and *Shape* magazines.

When asked why she invented the new 12-Minute Total-Body Workout, Joyce replied: "Time. As much as I love working out, I just can't afford to make it my life, and neither can most people with careers, families, etc. As my career began to develop, I found that I could no longer spare four or five hours a week to keep in shape—so I had to come up with a program that would get the job done with maximum efficiency and minimal time investment. I combined what I learned in the martial arts about isometric pressure and dynamic tension and what I learned from bodybuilders about muscle isolation and the split routine, and found that I could achieve a tight, toned body in minutes a day rather than hours a day. And the only sacrifice I had to make was to have smaller muscles than before. That was fine with me, since most people like smaller muscles anyway."

Joyce has been a guest on many national and local television shows. Among them are: "The Oprah Winfrey Show," "Hour Magazine," "Cable News Network," and "The Morning Show"; "Best Talk in Town" in New York, "Kelley and Company" in Detroit, and "Good Day" in Washington. She lives in Wantagh, New York, with her sixteen-year-old daughter, Marthe Simone.

Index